The Spiritual Healing of Traditional Thailand

C. Pierce Salguero

author of Encyclopedia of Thai Massage and A Thai Herbal

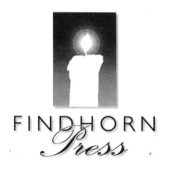

FINDHORN
Press

First published by Findhorn Press in 2006

ISBN 1-84409-072-8

British Library Cataloguing-in-Publication Data.
A Catalogue Record for this book is available from the British Library

Edited by Kate Keogan
Layout by C. Pierce Salguero
Cover Design by Thierry Bogliolo

Published by

Findhorn Press
305a The Park, Findhorn
Forres IV36 3TE, Scotland, UK
Tel 01309-690582 - Fax 01309-690036
info@findhornpress.com

www.findhornpress.com

CONTENTS

This book is dedicated to my teacher,
the late Ajahn Sintorn Chaichakan,
who passed away in 2005.
As the masters of the elder generations leave us,
may we be worthy to carry forth the jewels of wisdom
they have shared with us
in a spirit of *metta* and universal compassion.

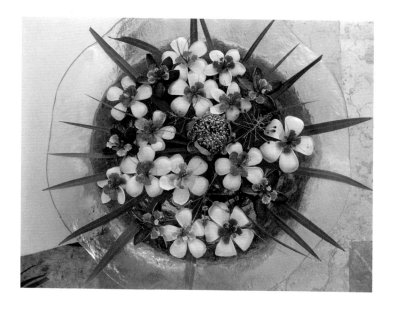

INTRODUCTION

The Circle of Life[1]

One of the primary teachings of traditional Thai medicine, and one of its most important insights, is the Circle of Life. This description of life says that three essences are always present: body, *citta*, and energy. In this formula, body means the physical structure, the atoms and molecules that make up the material self. Citta, often translated as mind-heart, is a word used to refer to the internal self, the inner processes which are not visible or directly measurable from the outside but which are real to each of us in our own subjective experience. Energy, in this system, is the force that animates both the body and the citta, linking them together.

In traditional Thai medicine, each of these essences is given equal weight, and it is said that all three must be present, balanced, and healthy in order for life to continue optimally. As the three are interconnected, injury, disease, or imbalance in one area naturally

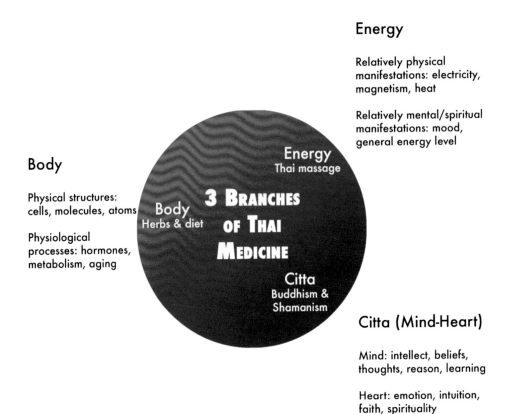

Energy

Relatively physical manifestations: electricity, magnetism, heat

Relatively mental/spiritual manifestations: mood, general energy level

Body

Physical structures: cells, molecules, atoms

Physiological processes: hormones, metabolism, aging

Citta (Mind-Heart)

Mind: intellect, beliefs, thoughts, reason, learning

Heart: emotion, intuition, faith, spirituality

The three branches of Thai medicine include therapies for the body, energy, and citta. As all diseases affect all three essences, so medicine must address all holistically.

leads to problems in the others. For example, if one is subjected to bodily injury, this theory says that mental imbalance (such as depression or fear) and lowered energy levels will result. Likewise, if one's mind and heart are not balanced, this will lead to energetic imbalance and disease in the body. Finally, if one's energy levels falter, this will lead to both mental and physical lethargy. Because disease originating in any of the three essences soon leads to imbalance in the others, traditional Thai medicine addresses these three essences equally and simultaneously.

In traditional Thai medicine hospitals, the Circle of Life is addressed within the same facility, under the same roof. At the Shivagakomarpaj Traditional Medicine Hospital, for example, there is a main building that houses all of the massage and herbal activity. To the right, you have the educational facilities where students learn traditional medicine. To the left are the herbal saunas, which provide herbal inhalation therapy. In the center of it all is the altar (see photos in Chapters 3 and 4).

The patient who is sick and comes for healing will first stop at the altar for meditation and offerings, and then go for their massage. After the massage they will go to the sauna to detoxify and sweat out impurities, and then to the herbalist for a consultation. They will finish once again at the altar before leaving. Thus, the whole Circle of Life is located all in one place, and all the medical specialists work together with the same holistic mindset.

The Spiritual Healing of Traditional Thailand

This book is the third in a three-part series on traditional Thai medicine that explores these three essences. The first title, *A Thai Herbal*, discussed therapies of the body: herbal and dietary medicine affecting the human organism at the physiological level. The second book, *The Encyclopedia of Thai Massage,* detailed the practices of Thai bodywork (called *nuad boran* in Thai), a system of massage which deals primarily with energy lines, yoga stretches, and pressure points designed to stimulate the body's energy flow.

This current book is about the citta, the mind and the heart. In traditional Buddhist language, this one word, citta, is used to mean both intellect and emotions at the same time. Unlike our own Western philosophy that has emphasized the difference between the mind and heart (or left-brain and right-brain, or thought and intuition), Buddhist philosophy sees these two as part of the same process, an inner self or consciousness that is not separated into different functions.

An over-used but helpful word to describe the practices of the citta is "spirituality," and the techniques which work on the citta "spiritual healing." In the Thai model, because body, energy, and citta are interlinked, working with the citta is important to overall health and well-being both before and after illness strikes — both for patients and practitioners. Thus, this book will discuss Thai ideas for both recovering from and preventing imbalance of the citta.

Thai spiritual healing is a fascinating multi-cultural heritage with many influences, and is part of what makes Thailand such a colorful and exciting place. In Thailand, because of its unique history, spiritual practices revolve mostly around Buddhist and indigenous animist traditions. However, at the end of the day, the message of the Circle of Life is not dependent on the practice of any one religious tradition. Many cultures have developed similar theories to fit their own cultural needs, and we can as well.

In this book, I wish to introduce the reader to a wide gamut of Thai spiritual life, from Buddhist meditation, to beliefs in spirits, to magical tattoos, and more. This book is intended, however, to be much more than just a review of a few techniques. In the process, I hope to spark an interest in you to want to read more — and perhaps even to experience some of these practices for yourself. With this in mind, I have provided additional resources and reading at the end of each chapter for future follow-up. Many of these are available through our website (www.taomountain.org).

A Comparison with Other Cultures

The chart on the next page draws parallels between the traditional healing practices of Thailand, India, and China, as well as with the modern West. I believe there are common threads in all four of these medical traditions, and we can see the Circle of Life at work in all.

In India, yoga is the energy discipline. The traditional reason for practicing yoga is to energize certain chakras (energy centers) in the body and to increase energy flow. In India there is also the

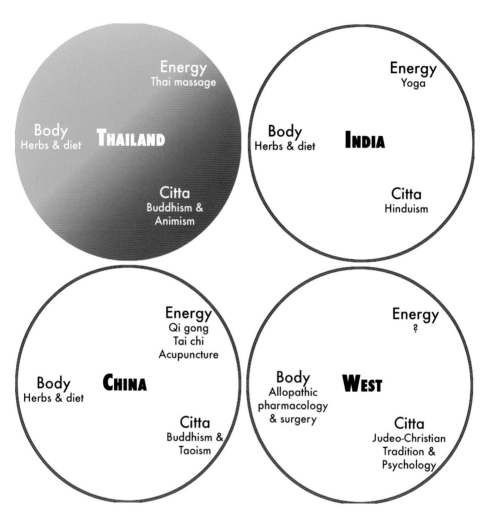

A comparison of the medical systems of four cultures.

body component, Ayurvedic herbs and diet. There is also the citta, or mental-spiritual component, which for India comes mostly from Hinduism, and includes practices such as meditation and chanting.

In China, acupuncture is an energy practice, as are qi gong and tai chi. The body practice in China is the discipline of herbal medicine and dietary theory. China's citta practice comes from the spiritual traditions of both Mahayana Buddhism and Taoism.

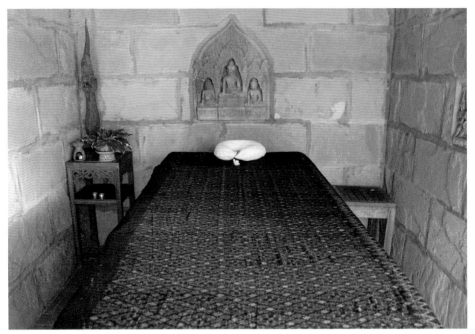

The setting for the practice of Thai medicine always includes elements of Buddhist tradition. This is a spa in Koh Samui.

In the West, most of the standard allopathic practices—such as surgery, physical therapy, and pharmaceutical medicine—concentrate predominantly on the body. Even while treating mental disorders, modern pharmaceutical medicine likes prescribes drugs which act on the physical body. However, not all Western medicine is focused on the chemical structure of the organism. There is also a well-developed science devoted to the citta, namely psychology. A therapist may encourage a patient to talk through problems effectively without ever resorting to treating the body on the chemical level. There is also a strong presence in the West of Judeo-Christian tradition, and religious practice (in whatever form it takes) helps many people to heal the citta.

The field of energy, however, is the one area that Western medicine typically leaves out. Perhaps we seek our energetic stimulation at the gym, and this is why we tend to enjoy working out so much. Perhaps

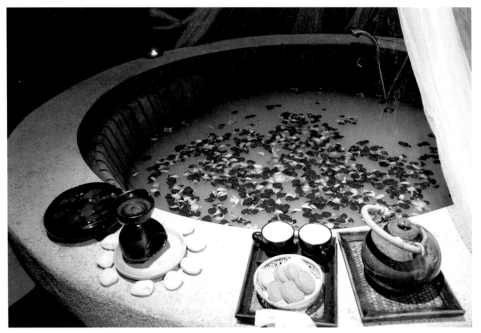

A hot herbal bath combines herbal inhalation therapy, medicinal teas, and a soothing environment. This treatment – or an herbal sauna – usually follows a Thai massage to provide treatment for all three essences.

this can also explain the popularity of yoga, tai chi, qi gong, reiki, martial arts, and even Thai massage in our culture. Even though we have yet to develop a Western medical science focused on energy, researchers have begun to look at electromagnetism as a useful healing technology. I believe that this field of medicine will continue to grow, filling the current void in our scientific understanding of energetic medicine.

Unlike in the Asian traditions, however, in the West, even when we find the three branches of medicine, these are normally quite antagonistic towards each other. It is true that you can find hospitals which include both a chapel and psychological services under the same roof and a more accepting approach to alternative techniques like acupuncture, but these practices have yet to be fully integrated. We are still a long way from MDs prescribing a visit to the herbalist or the priest!

The so-called holistic health movement has not historically been part of the solution either. Up until the present, allopathic doctors and holistic practitioners seldom have worked together to understand each other's perspectives. In the best case scenario, these communities have tolerated each other. In the worst cases, the two camps have been at war, the holistic community arguing that allopathic medicine is too aggressive and the allopathic medical community arguing that complementary medicine is bogus. Neither values the other's contribution to healthcare, so the stand-off continues.

While this situation has seen some notable improvement in recent years as Asian medical techniques gain popularity in some medical circles, there still is much work to do. Only through dialogue between Western medical professionals and holistic practitioners and through mutual understanding of the importance each plays in the field can this important work be done.

The important message of Thai medicine is that these three fields of healing — the physical, the energetic, and the spiritual — must be given equal weight and equal attention. All diseases or disorders affect all three essences, and thus all diseases require all three types of healing. All three types of healing must therefore be considered central to the field of medicine. This is the radical message of the Circle of Life: mental and emotional wellbeing are not incidental to physical health, but are an integral and necessary part of it. Or, to put it slightly differently: spirituality *is* medicine, and any medicine is not truly medicine unless it includes the spiritual.

End Notes

1. The Circle of Life philosophy presented here is one of the primary teachings in the courses of the Shivagakomarpaj Traditional Medicine Hospital in Chiang Mai, northern Thailand. This facility is one of the foremost schools of traditional Thai medicine in the country, and a healthcare facility which preserves the traditional model in the heart of a modern city. More information about this hospital is presented in Chapter 8.

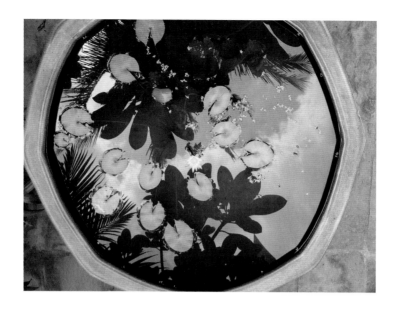

—1—

THAI BUDDHISM

Buddhism has become one of the most widely-practiced religious traditions in global history, and has fueled the production of magnificent art, architecture, and other cultural wonders from its earliest times. It has also become one of the most relevant spiritual practices of the modern day due to its message of tolerance, peace, and harmony. Historically, Buddhism has emphasized personal liberation through compassion and wisdom, while eschewing dogmatism, fanaticism, and violence. This tradition runs deep in the veins of Thailand, and any discussion of Thai spirituality must begin here.

Before it branched into the more elaborate and esoteric Mahayana schools of Tibet, China, and Japan, Buddhism was a simple spiritual path with a strong ethical code and a focus on meditation. This early

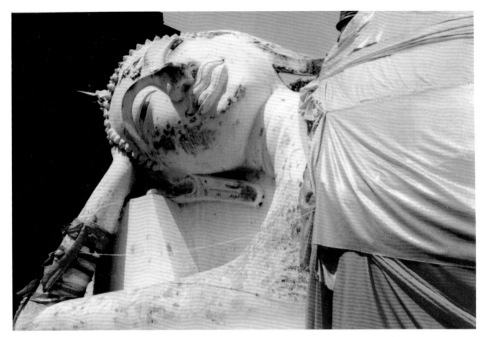

Saffron-clad reclining Buddha at Ayudhya, ancient capital of the Siamese kingdom.

form of Buddhism — preserved in Southeast Asian countries such as Thailand, Burma, Laos, and Sri Lanka — is known as the *Theravada* (Teachings of the Elders). This is the oldest form of this religion, most closely related to the original teachings of the historical Buddha. (This school of Buddhism is sometimes referred to as *Hinayana* by Tibetan and Chinese Buddhists, but this is a derogatory term meaning the "Lesser Vehicle," and it should be avoided.)

The founder of Buddhism, Siddhatta Gotama, is thought to have died around 486 BC. He is said to have been a prince who rejected the wealthy life of the palace in favor of becoming a wandering ascetic. Although this was a common lifestyle in ancient India, the Buddha discovered certain truths through meditation that were unknown to his contemporaries, and began to teach — first just to his ascetic companions, but then attracting a larger following.

Theravada Buddhism is based on a canon composed as early as

the fourth century BC, although it was not written down until at least 200 years later when it was recorded in the Pali language. The first part of this canon, the *Suttapitaka*, or basket of stories, is said to preserve the Buddha's sermons and conversations, as well as many stories about his life. A second section, the *Vinayapitaka* or basket of discipline, preserves the Buddhist monastic code, while a third basket, the *Abhidhammapitaka*, preserves a detailed compendium of Buddhist philosophy.

Despite the fact that the Pali texts have been fixed for the better part of the last 2000 years, Theravada Buddhism has nonetheless been a flexible living tradition. Buddhists the world over have always interpreted their religious faith in the light of local traditions, and Theravada Buddhism, too, has developed into a multitude of local variations. While these different schools have not taken on as much Hindu or Chinese influence as the Mahayana, Southeast Asian Buddhism is colored by the shamanic and animist elements of the region's pre-Buddhist traditions. Thai religion thus revolves around a blend of Theravada Buddhism and indigenous beliefs which are much older. These two traditions have coexisted and blended together to the point that they are inseparable today. This book will thus approach Thai spiritual healing traditions from both of these angles.

While he is usually deified in other forms of Buddhism, Theravadins (practitioners of the Theravada) believe that the historical Buddha, Siddhatta Gotama, was really just a man. The Theravada says that he did not achieve anything supernatural himself, or rely on any gods or divine powers to achieve salvation. The Buddha's enlightenment was a human achievement and lies within the realm of possibility for anyone. Thus Buddhist philosophy is ultimately humanistic: the practitioner is asked to do none other than fully embody humanity's highest potential, using the Buddha's teachings as a tool for achieving this goal.

The Buddha's teachings are eminently practical. He did not advocate dogmatic adherence to specific philosophies or beliefs, but rather advised his followers to accept nothing on faith, but pursue truth for themselves wherever it leads. The tradition of Theravada Buddhism emphasizes understanding oneself—the whole being, including the physical and the mental, which as we already have seen are inseparably intertwined. Through meditation practices that provide insight into the inner workings of the mind and body, practitioners come to understand the self and its relationship to the greater universe.

Theravada Buddhism holds that the path is one that everyone must walk alone, and that no one can carry your weight for you as you make your way through *samsara* (the endless cycle of birth and rebirth). Philosophically, Theravada Buddhism is fascinating in that it is the only major religion that is actually agnostic on the point of the existence of deities. There is no supreme deity in Buddhism, no creator god or savior figure: the ultimate truth is emptiness and selflessness.

Some deities (in Thai called *thewada*) do appear in popular Pali stories, and the Buddha also confronts beings who are personifications of evil (such as Mara). But a radically different interpretation of these deities and demons is presented: gods are considered to be higher reincarnations than humans and demons are lower, but all are, like us, still subject to suffering, death, and rebirth. Like us, these beings are doomed to be reborn again and again in the endless cycle. Gods are only different from us in that they get to live out their current lifetime in glorious heavens, while we have to live down on earth. The ideal Buddhist is not tempted by anything offered in the realm of gods or demons because he or she knows that it will not last and that even gods eventually suffer and die. Therefore, he or she seeks that which is beyond death and rebirth, total escape from samsara into nirvana, or emptiness.

Theravada Buddhist tradition holds that nirvana is one of the great "imponderables": until we become enlightened, we cannot know what it is. Thus, anything we say about it is only speculation, and is therefore a waste of time. However, rather than ask for our blind faith, the Buddha said that we should not take anything said by him or by other religious leaders as truth. We should accept something as

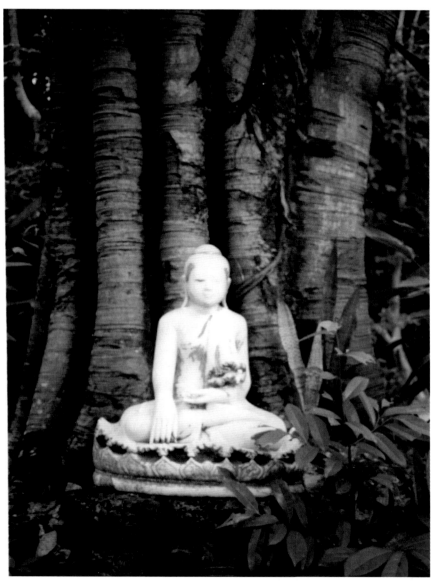

A Buddha statue under a tree is symbolic of Sidhatta Gotama achieving enlightenment under the Bodhi tree. Notice the earth-touching gesture with the right hand. This is reminiscent of the Buddha's confrontation with Mara, the personification of evil. Mara challenged the Buddha, asking him what gave him the audacity to think he could become enlightened. In silence, the Buddha answered by touching the earth to call her to bear witness to the countless previous lives he had lived helping people, building the enormous stock of merit required to become a Buddha. (Wat Pah Nanachat)

truth only after we have experienced it for ourselves. So rather than endless philosophizing about the intricate workings of the universe, the immediate priority is to work on meditation techniques to help us along in this direction. Thus it is practice, not dogma, that is Buddhism's primary concern.

Making Merit

The foundation of practice in Buddhism is morality. The Buddhist idea of karma is practically a household word now, most people being familiar with its concept of cause and effect. Essentially, karma says that for every cause there is a consequence: for every act of good or evil we commit, we plant seeds of good or evil that will affect our future, either in this life or in the next.

All Buddhist traditions I know of emphasize following the Five Precepts as the basic moral code. In Thailand, these precepts are undertaken by all Buddhists as lifetime vows:

1. To refrain from killing any living being
2. To refrain from taking what is not given
3. To refrain from sexual misconduct (for non-monastics this is mainly rape, incest, and adultery; for monks, this is total celibacy)
4. To refrain from unwholesome or false speech
5. To refrain from intoxicants (any substances which cloud, impair, or transform the mind, including alcohol, marijuana, other drugs, etc.). In monasteries across Asia, caffeine and sugar are usually not considered intoxicants, although opinions differ from place to place on tobacco.

The idea behind these five precepts is to refrain from activities that injure yourself or others and to maintain clarity and peacefulness in life. By following these precepts, a practitioner avoids accumulating "bad karma" and generates merit, instead.

One of the common ways that Thai Buddhist laypeople make merit is through almsgiving. Unlike their Mahayana and Tibetan counterparts, Theravada monks are not allowed to support themselves financially.

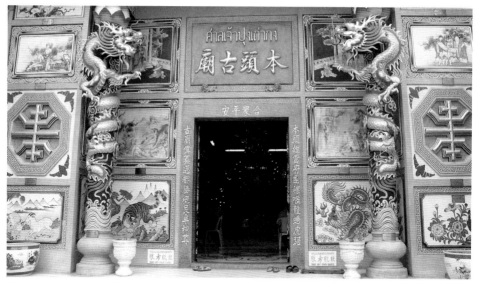

Chinese temples like this one are found all over Thailand, especially in larger cities, but these serve Chinese populations, and follow Chinese Buddhism or Taoism. Chinese Buddhism belongs to the Mahayana tradition, a school of Buddhism which evolved 500-1000 years following the Buddha's death and which is very different from Theravada. (Bangkok)

They must completely renounce all wealth, all income, bank accounts, and possessions. Traditionally, monks are prohibited from even touching money, and thus must rely entirely on the generosity of the community and sustain themselves by collecting alms.

Alms-rounds, or *pindabat*, is a highly ritualized part of Buddhist life, and, as a daily routine, it is a constant reminder to both monks and laypeople alike of the interdependent relationship between the town and the temple. This ancient daily ritual seems more fitting in the countryside than in the busy streets of cities like Bangkok but, as a rule, urban Thais are as devout as those in the provinces.

Monks are not allowed to ask for donations. A monk simply is supposed to walk with his bowl, and be satisfied with whatever is put into it. Alms mostly consist of offerings of food and drinking

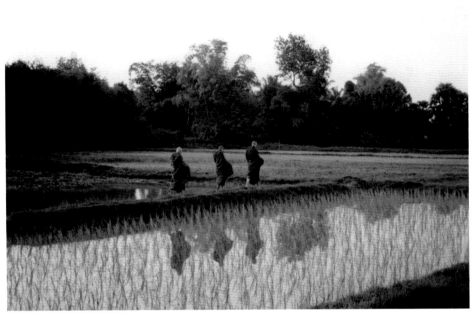

Monks on pindabat, or alms-rounds, in rural northeast Thailand.

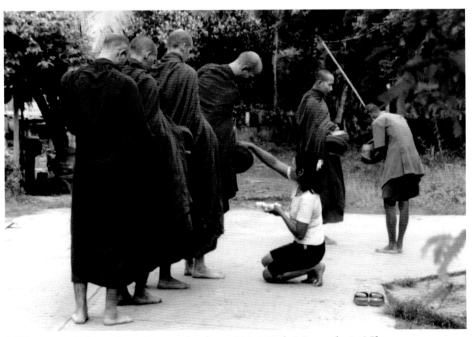

Villagers giving alms to monks from Wat Pah Nanachat, Ubon Rachathani.

water, but may also include religious items like lotus flowers, incense, and candles, or other essentials like soap, laundry detergent, and toothpaste — all the necessities that the renunciates cannot buy due to their vow of poverty. Anyone who wishes to make merit can donate food by approaching the monk, bowing, and placing gifts into the metal bowl. Many rural people bring out home-made dishes, but in the cities it is more common to purchase items from street vendors. Throughout the streets of any Thai city, morning stalls do brisk business by selling alms to the devout.

Pindabat is a religious ritual, and monks do not engage in conversation while collecting their food. It is unusual that they address or be addressed by the donors. Sometimes, the layperson will mumble a prayer while giving alms, but never direct words towards the monk. More often than not, the hour or two passes in complete silence. Another tradition of the pindabat is that monks do not wear shoes. Whether they slog through knee-deep rice paddies or trod the cement sidewalks of the city, monks on alms-rounds typically go barefoot. The purpose of this solemnity is to remind the laypeople and the monks of the religious nature of the exchange. This is not the same as giving a few coins to a beggar at a bus station; it is a ceremony thousands of years old that transcends both the giver and the receiver.

After completing their appointed rounds, monks return to their monasteries to eat. Each monk typically collects much more food than any one person could consume in a day. All of the food and toiletries collected are shared among the monastic community according to their needs, and any leftovers are often distributed to the poor in a daily soup-kitchen sponsored by the temple. Any food still left after that is given to the stray cats and dogs that have learned to hang around the temples in the afternoon.

The *Wat* and Society

In Theravada cultures, there is an important relationship between the *wat* (or the temple) and the surrounding village or neighborhood. The laity helps to support the monks materially and the temple financially. The monks on the other hand provide the community with a source of advice, assistance, and spiritual teaching, and they perform all of society's required rituals.

The temple is also a community center that often includes various charities. Almost all temples provide the area's hungry with a source of free meals. Many offer education to monks and novices—the Buddhist equivalent of parochial school. Temples are involved with children's groups, with community development, agricultural projects, and other local issues. In the 1980s and 90s, with the AIDS rate rising, many celibate monks found themselves ironically involved with sex education and family-planning programs as well.

The wats have kept Buddhist religious traditions alive despite the relentless pace of modernization in the past two decades precisely through this growing involvement in modern life. Much of life— whether in the city or the village—is centered around the temples. Despite the onslaught of Western influence and technology, religion is still an inseparable part of every-day existence in Thailand.

Naturally, Thai Buddhism is fighting an up-hill battle against modern secularism and other forces that threaten to dilute the traditions, but Theravada Buddhism still lies at the heart of Thailand today. There are still over 30,000 temples in operation in the country, probably more Buddhist temples per capita than in any other country in the world, and this network remains undoubtedly the most prominent social force.

Obviously, Buddhism is not an oasis exempt from the proclivities of human nature, and the monkhood suffers as much as any other segment of society at the hands of the greedy and the manipulative. But these examples are the exceptions, not the norm. The majority of Theravada monks have forsaken the so-called worldly life, including owning money and possessions, in order to pursue full-time religious education and spiritual training.

Theravada Buddhism treats the journey to Nirvana as a personal quest, and each monk is meant to devote himself whole-heartedly to this path. In actuality, most city monks don't do much meditation.

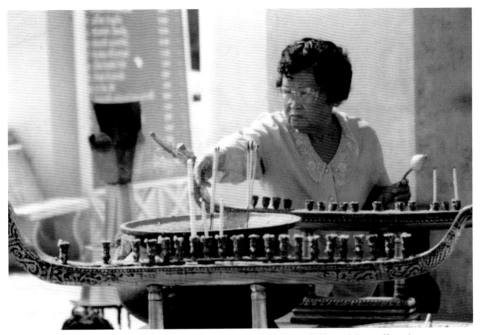

Lighting candles and incense in honor of the Buddha. (Ayudhya)

They study the Pali texts, teach, and perform ceremonies. But there are many forest temples in Thailand, Burma, and across Southeast Asia that specialize in meditation, and teach techniques that, even today, produce *arhats* (or enlightened beings).

The majority of the practicing laity, on the other hand, is made up of women, who participate in all aspects of religious life aside from ordination in the monkhood. Women have not had the opportunity to become nuns since the female lineage died out around 900 AD. However, it is typically women who attend meditation retreats, lectures, and temple events. While ordained men and boys spend much of their time on performing rituals and studying religious texts as dictated by their formal requirements, women, on the other hand, often are the ones doing the serious personal practice.

Visiting a Thai Temple

While investigating Thai temples, I have found the monks to be very

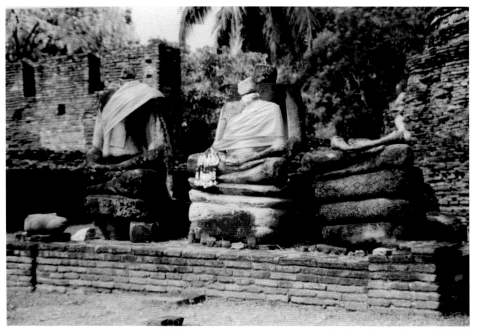

Buddha statues from the Ayudhya period. These statues have lost their heads due to the poaching of art collectors. Keeping Thailand's cultural heritage intact has been an ongoing challenge in the face of criminal activity and international art smuggling.

friendly, curious, and receptive to visitors. They are usually well-educated, and eager to practice their English by giving a tour or answering questions. Some of the wats offer free accommodations for visitors with a sincere interest in Buddhism (Theravada temples always offer their services free of charge), although it's usually just a spot on the hard wood floors of the monks' quarters!

September is a particularly good time to be visiting temples. The rains retreat (or *pansa*) is sort of like a Buddhist Lent that lasts from the end of July to the end of October. This is an especially important period for laypeople and monks alike. During this time, laypeople often observe certain moral restrictions such as refraining from sex or meat, and participate in charitable acts and religious ceremonies to make merit. Monks also observe additional austerities during these months, typically concentrating on serious study and meditation. In most of Thailand, there is a tradition that a young man is not considered worthy for marriage unless he has spent at least one pansa ordained as a monk, so this is a period of time when the number of ordinations across the country swells. A small monastery of several dozen monks can become home to hundreds of temporary monks, mostly young teenagers, during the rains.

Any time of year, the best day to visit a Thai temple is on *wan phra*, Thailand's equivalent to the Sabbath. This is not a particular day of the week, but is determined by the phases of the moon. Laypeople can be found on any weekday praying and making offerings within the temple grounds, but on wan phra, the crowds at the temples are larger, and the evening ceremonies are especially well-attended.

The typical wan phra ceremony is in the evening. Laypeople and monks prostrate before the Buddha statues, and sit on the ground in rows to listen. The half-hour service involves several chants led by the abbot or senior monk, and is punctuated by stretches of silent meditation, a small melodic gong marking the transition from one segment to the next.

The chants are familiar words all Thais have heard countless times throughout life: pieces of scripture, codes of conduct, professions of faith such as those described in the third chapter. The assembled crowd knows when to bow their heads, when to *wai* (make a prayer gesture), and when to prostrate. The visiting foreigner, who will undoubtedly be a bit lost, is welcome to sit and participate, or just watch.

Additional Reading

If you are interested in Buddhism, you may want to consult the following titles:

Maguire, Jack. Essential Buddhism: A Complete Guide to Beliefs and

Practices. Atria, 2001. – This is the best introduction to Buddhism I know of. It is very engaging and highly readable.

Gethin, Rupert. The Foundations of Buddhism. Oxford University Press, 1998. – This is a wonderful and well-respected introductory academic text to Theravada Buddhism. While it is not specific to Thailand, it details many of the doctrinal foundations of Thai Buddhism.

Gombrich, Richard. Theravada Buddhism: A Social History from Ancient Benares to Modern Colombo. London: Routledge, 1988. – This is a classic work on Theravada Buddhism, well-known to any scholar of this religion, and is a must-read for anyone interested in the history of Thai Buddhist traditions.

Bhikkhu Ñanamoli and Bhikkhu Bodhi. The Middle Length Discourses of the Buddha: A Translation of the Majjhima Nikaya. Somerville, MA: Wisdom Publications, 1995. – I highly recommend Bhikkhu Bodhi, as he has translated or contributed to translation of many wonderful collections of the Buddhist canon, the *suttas*. The Middle-Length Discourses are the place to start for the first-time reader. These suttas are classics of world literature, and are indispensable for a deeper understanding of all forms of Buddhism, Theravada in particular.

www.accesstoinsight.org – This website contains loads of information on Theravada Buddhism, translation of Buddhist scripture, and lots of links to related organizations.

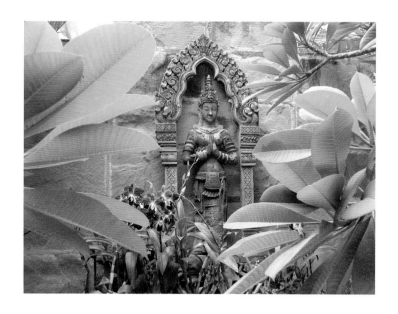

—2—

BUDDHIST MEDITATION

The Eightfold Noble Path

The Buddha's main teaching is the Eightfold Noble Path, which he proclaimed is the path to enlightenment, the fulfillment of the highest human potential. The steps on this path are not sequential, and are to be practiced all at the same time:

Path of Wisdom
    1. Right understanding—understanding the motivation for spiritual practice
    2. Right thought—bringing your thoughts towards beneficial things, and not focusing on negative or unwholesome thoughts and emotions

Path of Morality
    3. Right speech—refraining from lying, slander, gossip, and harsh talk

4. Right action—following the five precepts

5. Right livelihood—engaging in a livelihood which is in line with the five precepts and which benefits self and other beings (examples of unacceptable livelihood include butcher, drug dealer, alcohol sales, military, etc.)

Path of Meditation

6. Right effort—having a resolute drive to meditate

7. Right mindfulness—being continually mindful of the body and mind in all of your actions and thoughts

8. Right concentration—developing the ability to focus in meditation to penetrate to deep levels of understanding

As you can see from this list, meditation makes up a large part of the Buddhist path, and this is the focus of the present chapter.

Starting a Meditation Practice

The setting for meditation practice should be a quiet comfortable place, ideally one that is reserved for this activity and is removed from places like kitchens and offices that we use for every-day life. You may wish to set up an altar to create a sacred space devoted to your meditation practice, and instructions on setting up a Thai altar are given in the next chapter.

The classic meditation posture is sitting cross-legged on a cushion on the floor, but it is perfectly fine to sit in another position if this is uncomfortable. Ideally, you want to keep yourself erect rather than slouching, which can cause drowsiness, so if you are using a chair, use a straight-backed dining room chair rather than an easy chair or couch.

The two meditations described in this chapter follow a similar pattern. Meditation requires first and foremost the cultivation of attention. Our minds are used to flitting and fluttering about from one thought to another all day long, and are not accustomed to sustained concentration for longer than a few seconds. So, the first step in any meditation practice will be to develop the ability to concentrate for

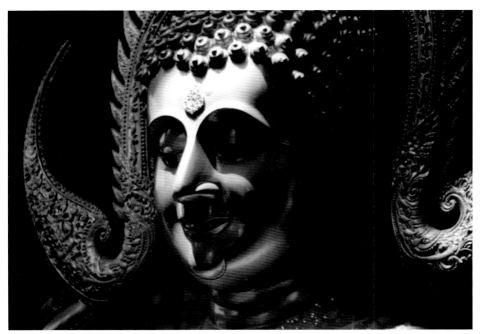

This golden Buddha in Ayudhya, like all Theravada icons, is intended to capture the serenity of nirvana. Note the classic Buddhist iconographical details: the elongated ears, the slight smile, the half-closed eyes, the urna *(third-eye mark), the snail-shell curled hair, and the* mandorla, *a type of halo intended to convey the light of wisdom.*

longer and longer periods of time on a single thing.

This "single thing" is called the object of meditation. In practice, your object can be any number of different things, and the Buddha was known to give different objects to different people depending on their abilities and personalities. Today there are a fixed number of acceptable meditation objects based on Pali texts. However, Theravada Buddhist meditations all have one thing in common: the object is always real. The truths that meditation works with are quite simple, and often escape our notice on a daily basis. You will notice

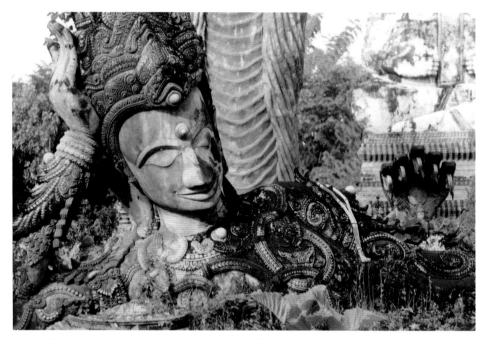

A reclining statue in a garden at Wat Khaek in Nong Khai, northern Thailand.

that the meditations below work with breath, with the body, and with the mind. These truths are always with us, and always available because they are a part of us.

Mindfulness of Breathing Meditation

Here a monk, having gone into the forest, or to the root of a tree, or to an empty place, sits down cross-legged, holding his body erect, having established mindfulness before him. Mindfully he breathes in, mindfully he breathes out. Breathing in a long breath, he knows that he breathes in a long breath, and breathing out a long breath, he knows that he breathes out a long breath. Breathing in a short breath, he knows that he breathes in a short breath, and breathing out a short breath, he knows that he breathes out a short breath. He trains himself, thinking: "I will breathe in, conscious of the whole body." He trains himself, thinking: "I will breathe out, conscious of the whole body."[1]

Mindfulness of breathing (called *anapanasati*), is one of the most popular and most simple Buddhist meditations, and is found all over the Buddhist world. There are several mentions of this practice in the Pali canon, including an entire text entitled *Anapanasati Sutta*. In almost every instance, this practice is said to be among the most effective and beneficial meditation practices in the Buddhist tradition. Many schools of Buddhism focus entirely on breathing meditation, and it is said that this practice alone is sufficient to bring enlightenment.

To practice mindfulness of breathing meditation, you must choose a spot for your attention right on the tip of your nose by your nostrils. Next, sit quietly and breathe normally. Without modifying the pace or intensity of your inhalations and exhalations, simply try to remain aware of that spot on your nose with each breath. Notice the breath passing over that spot on your nose, and notice the quality of each breath. Is it long? Short?

Start with shorter periods of time (15-30 minutes) and work up to longer (45-60). One of the most important parts of the practice of meditation is to see how long you can maintain your chosen object in your awareness. Of course at first your mind will wander. (If you're like me, you'll spend 99% of your meditation time daydreaming and thinking about everything other than your object!) With time and patience, however, this wandering will decrease.

If you need to count your breaths in order to help you maintain attention when first starting out, you can do so. See if you can count to 10 breath cycles without losing track, and then start over. Another common practice in Thailand is to breathe out while silently thinking the word "Buddha." Both counting and reciting the Buddha's name are only tools to help with concentration to get you started. You should as soon as possible change over to silent breathing without any assistance from any type of verbalization.

Meditation is a lot like learning any new skill. It takes practice, perseverance, and effort. Like learning the piano, it's a lot more effective to do a bit every day rather than a whole lot once in a while. Unlike learning the piano, though, you don't have benchmarks to easily measure your progress.

You can not force this to happen, but eventually, naturally, you may come to the point that you can fix your attention on your breathing, and remain aware of each breath passing in and out for longer periods of time. With this ability, you will find that your thoughts are becoming increasingly quiet, and that you are becoming increasingly aware of the inner workings of the mind.

The insights that will reveal themselves to you at this time, according to the Buddha's teachings, are the three characteristics of all existence:

1. *Anicca* (impermanence) — That which arises also passes away. Any event, situation, feeling, thought, etc., that you experience is bound to change with time. Nothing is ever permanent. You can see this great truth in your own meditation practice. Notice how every day leads to different experiences in your practice and how no two moments are ever alike. When you feel bored, emotional, stiff, or negative, notice how this soon fades away or changes into something else. Also notice how even wonderful feelings also disappear and change.

2. *Dukkha* (unsatisfactoriness) — If nothing is permanent, if follows that nothings bring us permanent happiness. Anything we accumulate or try to hold on to in order to make ourselves happy is bound to be unsatisfactory in the long run because it is bound to change or disappear. Buddhism teaches that there is no permanent blissfully happy state. Our lives are always in flux and flow.

3. *Anatta* (non-self) — If the above is true, then the only chance at happiness is for us to learn to accept and flow with the ever-changing phenomena all around us. When we realize that our best strategy is to openly accept life as an endless stream of ever-changing events, our own self-importance and attachment to ego begins to diminish.

Buddhism teaches that all notions of self are ultimately illusory.

Even if we believe these three principles as matters of philosophy, it is quite a different thing to actually experience them within our mind and body. But this is the purpose of anapanasati meditation. Of course, these insights will not just suddenly appear. They will gradually develop over many years of regular practice.

More likely, your beginning experiences will be full of frustration, false starts, and questions. When you reach a difficult point, you should do two things. First, remember that the entire point of the practice is to realize the three characteristics above, including the first one on the list, anicca, or change. Your meditation practice is — like all things — subject to change. It won't always be easy, and it won't always be blissful. Sometimes ugly memories, negative thoughts, and difficult emotions arise in meditation. Usually the things we want to hide from the most are the things that pop up first. It is important when this happens to treat these thoughts as you would treat all other thoughts that arise as the mind wanders: as soon as possible, set these down, and come back to the meditation object. No need to get frustrated, upset, angry, or emotional... just pick up where you left off and keep going.

The second thing you should do is consult a meditation teacher. You should realize that no one can learn meditation from a book without personalized guidance. These meditations are presented here in order to give you a taste and a starting point. If you find yourself interested in the meditations presented here, after experimenting a bit with them, find a reliable teacher who can help you to cultivate your new practice (see details at the end of this chapter).

Remember, though, when seeking out a teacher, to do your homework. In the Pali canon, the Buddha says, "Be an island unto yourself." In Theravada Buddhism, we seek a teacher not because they are some deity-like individual who is going to save us, but because they are able to teach us something of value — something with real and tangible benefit for us. Typically, monks and practicing Buddhists in Thailand spend 5 years with a teacher learning meditation techniques.

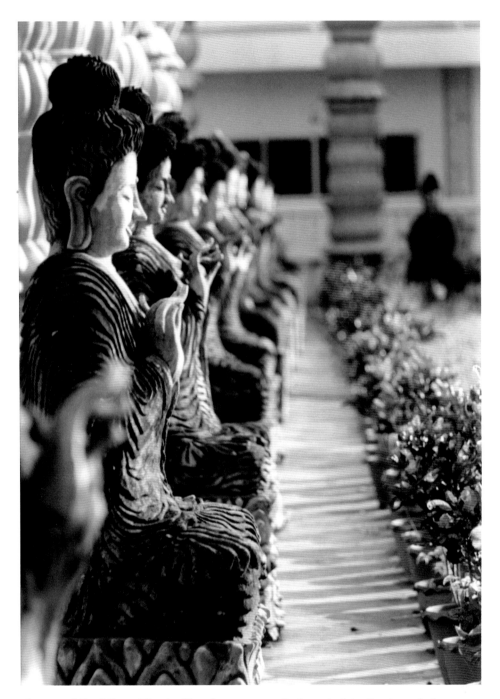

A row of Buddhas. Typically, these are each donated to the temple by a family or individual. (Nong Khai)

However, the student is always free to learn from other individuals as well, and to change their primary meditation technique at any time. The study of Buddhism should be practical, and the student should always place their own judgment at the top of the list of priorities.

Metta Meditation

Metta meditation is another important technique for the cultivation of both mental, and by extension, physical well-being. For most Buddhists, practice of the Buddhist path means cultivation of positive mental states such as compassion and mental clarity. Most Thais understand this in the context of merit, karma, and reincarnation. The more merit you have accumulated, the less bad karma, the better the next life will be.

They say that the wheel of rebirth has gone around so many times that every creature you meet has at one point or another been your mother, father, child, or teacher — or will be in the next life. Therefore, you should remember to cultivate compassion and goodwill towards all creatures, because we will meet them again and again in samsara. Many Westerners find reincarnation a difficult philosophy to accept, but even if we don't believe, we can still use the idea as a practical teaching tool.

How can we learn to meet everyone and every situation with goodwill? Every religion says "love thy neighbor," but in the rush of daily life this lesson is often completely forgotten. All too often, without even realizing it we find ourselves awash in negativity like anger, stress, anxiety, jealousy, etc., which hurt us both mentally and physically in the long run. Fortunately, Buddhism offers many different meditation tools, and one specifically given to help to curb negative states of mind.

One of the most common meditation practices in modern Theravada Buddhism is the active cultivation of positive mental states. This type of practice is designed to infiltrate our negative mental habits and plant messages of love and goodwill. It can be used to develop any of the four so-called *Brahma Viharas* (or Divine Abidings):

1. Loving kindness *(metta)* — the feeling that all beings are our friends and that we wish to benefit all through our actions.
2. Compassion *(karuna)* — the feeling of pity or sympathy for the suffering of other beings.
3. Sympathetic joy *(mudita)* — the feeling of joy (free from jealousy) for the happiness of other beings.
4. Equanimity *(upekkha)* — being unmoved by life's vicissitudes. Whatever comes your way, you react with equal calm and detachment.

The meditation I will present here is *metta-bhavana*, or the generation of loving kindness, but it can be modified for any of the above. This meditation operates along the lines of positive self-suggestions. Many people make the mistake of trying to *make* themselves feel something, and then feel self-conscious and stiff if they do not succeed. In practicing this technique, you should not force your feelings. Think of this meditation as a concentration exercise instead, and simply repeat the words over and over again. It is without trying that truly amazing things can happen.

I first started this meditation technique while staying at a monastery in Thailand. At first I felt foolish repeating these phrases to myself. But a monk I respected very much told me the following analogy. He said, most of us go through life with a mental habit pattern of negativity. Like a tape playing on an endless loop in our brain, our minds are constantly telling us to be unhappy. Even when we're not paying explicit attention to this tape, it still colors our every interaction in the background. The following meditation, he said, is simply changing that tape for one that says to be happy. If you practice this meditation for an hour, he told me, you'll have gained an hour of positive thoughts and an hour's rest from negative thoughts.

So, I decided to try it, and I practiced every day I was at the monastery. And within a very short period of time — no more than a few weeks — I found that these metta phrases were stuck in my head, repeating themselves subconsciously throughout the day. I also noticed that my heart felt lighter, and my outlook was more positive. And then, on one day, I felt waves of joy for no apparent reason as

I walked through the trees around the monastery. Since that time, I have realized that I benefit most from this practice when I do not try to achieve anything.

The lesson of this exercise is that the human mind is a creature of habit, and it can get stuck in a certain kind of thinking. If you need to break out of a pattern of thinking and replace it with something positive, this meditation can help.

I have written out below the phrases I was taught to use at the monastery, but there is no reason not to substitute your own if something else resonates more for you. The technique goes like this: close your eyes, and breathe naturally. Then, begin to repeat the phrases slowly in your mind. Let the phrases be your object of meditation. Again, start with shorter periods and work up. See how many times you can repeat them before you find your thoughts wandering. Whenever this happens, just pick back up where you left off and continue the repetitions. With time you will see that your concentration improves with practice, and your mind will be less and less distracted.

The idea with the cultivation of metta is to start with yourself, and gradually broaden out to a wider and wider group, ending with all sentient beings everywhere. If you have less time, you can stick to a few repetitions. I like to send metta to myself, the group I am sitting with, our friends and families, then all people everywhere, and then all other beings near and far, seen and unseen. If you have more time, though, you can develop more detailed meditations where you send metta to specific people or groups of people. Some meditations go on like this for an entire hour sending metta to countless people without ever repeating!

Metta Meditation

May I abide in well-being,
in freedom from hostility,
in freedom from ill-will,

in freedom from anxiety,
and may I maintain well-being in myself.
May I be released from all suffering,
and may I not be parted from the good fortune I have attained.

May we abide in well-being,
in freedom from hostility,
in freedom from ill-will,
in freedom from anxiety,
and may we maintain well-being in ourselves.
May we be released from all suffering,
and may we not be parted from the good fortune we have attained.

May all beings abide in well-being,
in freedom from hostility,
in freedom from ill-will,
in freedom from anxiety,
and may they maintain well-being in themselves.
May they be released from all suffering,
and may they not be parted from the good fortune they have attained.[2]

The Effects of Meditation

Practiced regularly, anapanasati and metta-bhavana meditation are said to lead to enlightenment by overcoming the Ten Fetters, or negative states of mind which should be eradicated at every opportunity...

1. Self-illusion—the belief that your ego is real
2. Ignorance—willfully causing negative mental states
3. Sensual craving—craving after objects which taste, smell, sound, feel, or look good
4. Ill-will—anger, hatred, jealousy, bitterness, etc.
5. Skepticism—doubt (especially self-doubt)
6. Restlessness—inability to sit still and concentrate
7. Conceit—self-centeredness

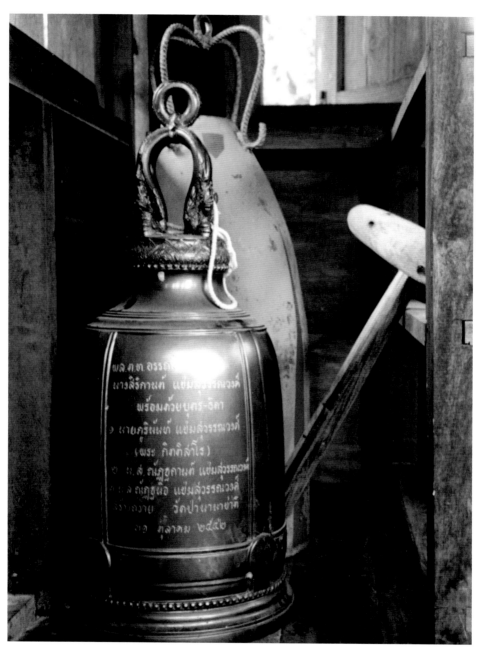

A moving example of metta in action, turning negativity into positivity: behind the bronze temple bell is a yellow and red bombshell found in a rural area after the Vietnam War. This bomb was emptied out and converted into a bell. It is rung daily to summon monks to meditation. (Wat Pah Nanachat, Ubon Rachathani)

8. Attachment to religion and rituals
9. Craving for material existence — desiring endless life on earth, or being afraid to die
10. Craving for non-material existence — desiring to die

... and to help generate the Ten Virtues, which should be cultivated at every opportunity:

1.   Generosity
2.   Morality
3.   Non-attachment
4.   Wisdom
5.   Energy
6.   Patience, tolerance, and forbearance
7.   Honesty
8.   Determination
9.   Loving kindness (metta)
10. Equanimity

Buddhism and Healing

Anyone who works in the healing professions in Thailand will attempt to bring the principles of Buddhism into their everyday work. Sometimes, this means participation in meditation retreats and other opportunities to learn techniques such as the ones just presented. Often, it is through ceremonies such as the *wai khru*, described in Chapter 4. Almost always, it means at least observing the five precepts. The fundamental point is that the Thai healer works to embody within themselves the principles of loving kindness and compassion, and to bring these into their work with patients. By cultivating positive mental states, and refraining from behavior that reinforces negative ones, healers can protect themselves from taking on detrimental negative energies, and have a healing effect on the individuals with whom they come in contact.

End Notes

1. Digha Nikaya ii.290. From *Walsche, Maurice. The Long Discourses of the Buddha: A Translation of the Digha Nikaya. Boston: Wisdom Publications, 1995*, p. 335-36.

2. *Saddhatissa, Ven. Dr. and Maurice Walshe. Chanting Book: Morning and Evening Puja and Reflections. Hertfordshire (UK): Amaravati Publications, 1994*, p. 41.

Additional Resources

If you are interested in meditation, you may want to consult the following titles:

Kornfield, Jack. Living Dharma: Teachings of Twelve Buddhist Masters. Boston: Shambhala, 1996. — This book is a wonderful introduction to 12 Buddhist teachers, half of whom were native to Thailand. Kornfield, a well-known meditation teacher himself, covers the breadth of teaching styles and meditation techniques taught in Theravada Buddhism. This is a great place to start for those interested in pursuing Thai Buddhism and meditation.

Hart, William. The Art of Living: Vipassana Meditation as taught by S.N. Goenka. San Francisco: Harper, 1987. — This is the best basic introduction to meditation I know of. It is fun, light, and very insightful. Goenka offers free 10-day Vipassana retreats world-wide, and is a highly respected Theravada Buddhist teacher.

Of course, at the end of the day, if you are really interested in learning about meditation, the best way to do so is to find a teacher and start a personal practice. To find a teacher in Theravada Buddhism, I suggest starting with the book by Jack Kornfield above. This book profiles some of the major meditation teachers of the past half century, many of whom have passed on, but whose students are now teaching their techniques. See which style you identify with, and seek it out. Many of these lineages now have websites and contacts all over the world.

You may also want to check out several Theravada monasteries which have meditation retreats in the West, including:

www.forestshangha.org — Wat Pah Nanachat is a traditional Thai monastery in the Forest Tradition. Founded by Thai meditation master Ajahn Chah in order to ordain a Western monkhood, this monastery provides a unique live-in experience for the most serious students of Buddhism (shaving heads and eyebrows required!). Other branch monasteries are also listed here, including Abhayagiri, a traditional Thai forest monastery in Northern California, and Amaravati, a traditional Thai forest monastery in England.

www.bhavanasociety.org — A traditional Theravada monastery in West Virginia, 2 hours from Washington DC. Retreats offered year-round on donation basis.

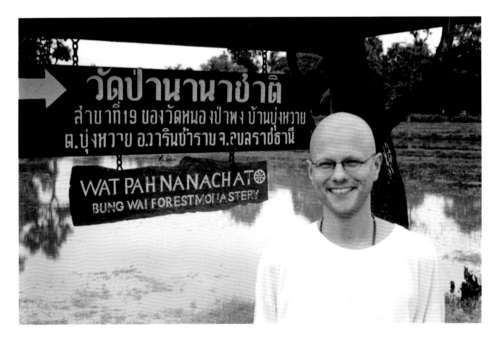

The author at the Wat Pha Nanachat monastery in Ubon Rachathani. Shaving the head and eyebrows is a requirement for ordination in Thai monasteries. Wat Pha Nanachat requires all visitors to take this step on the third day of their stay, to be sure that only serious students stick around!

www.dhamma.org – While not a monastery, S.N. Goenka's organization is run on a traditional model, and provides laypeople with the opportunity to participate in long retreats. This is a worldwide network of meditation centers, teaching the technique of Vipassana. See also their subdomain *vri.dhamma.org*, which contains links to research on Buddhism and psychology.

Note: Always remember the litmus test in Theravada Buddhism. If it is a traditional teaching, it should always be 100% free of charge. Authentic Theravada Buddhist teachers believe that it is hypocritical to charge people money to learn a technique of relieving suffering.

C. Pierce Salguero

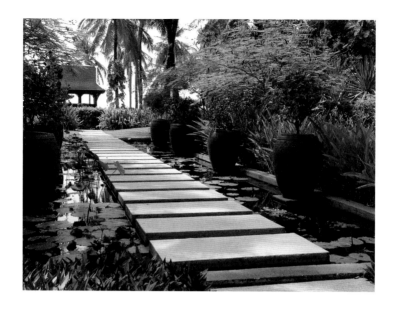

—3—

THE THAI ALTAR

Before venturing into the next two chapters focusing on some guidelines for the practice of Thai rituals, I'd like to offer a personal note. I know that what I am about to detail may seem archaic and irrelevant to some readers. Even if you recognize that these are very old Asian traditions and appreciate them as culturally important, these conventions still may seem strange or optional in a modern Western context where we have very few rituals that we still follow. However, having spent time in monasteries in Thailand where your every movement is subject to scrutiny and where there are many more regulations, and having stuck my foot in my mouth many a time when negotiating unfamiliar cultural territory, I can only offer you this bit of advice...

In my experience, the rules governing these ceremonies are initially difficult to understand but eventually become second nature. By this

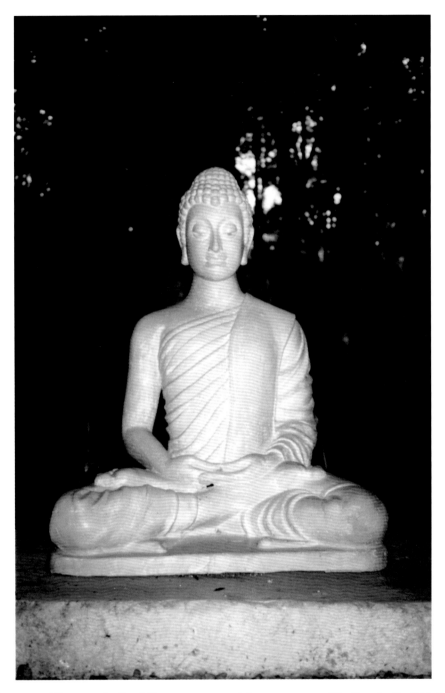

A serene Theravada Buddha statue presides over a meditation hall. (Wat Pah Nanachat Monastery, Ubon Rachathani)

time, you will hopefully see that these rules are not arbitrary, but are designed with one purpose in mind: to show respect and humility towards a tradition and a belief which is much larger than you.

When we are not merely outsiders studying Thai spirituality from afar but are starting to practice, we become part of the living fabric of this culture. In becoming a part of this tradition, we agree to learn to follow these rules in order to enter into a living relationship with this ancient lineage. We are also becoming the teachers and transmitters of the future, and if we neglect a part of this tradition, this part—which may have been carried for thousands of years—will become permanently lost. Therefore, these guidelines are, in my opinion, not optional but centrally important to the study and practice of Thai tradition.

I also honestly believe that one can come to enjoy these ritualized movements. Like the Japanese tea ceremony, or the movements of a martial art, the minute attention to detail can become a meditation in motion. Strict rules can be powerful tools to help us to become highly focused and attuned to our behavior, and can help us to cultivate mindfulness as we proceed with our daily tasks.

I truly enjoy performing the Thai ceremonies. It helps me to ground myself in the spirit of mindfulness and metta. It is also an opportunity for me to step outside of my self, my desires, and my daily routine, in order to tap into something much more ancient, more spiritual, and more meaningful than my common everyday life.

The Thai Buddha Icon

The altar is of central importance to the creation of a sacred space for the practice of Thai ceremonies. The typical Thai altar will display multiple items, and can include icons from other religions or traditions, including images from Hinduism, Mahayana Buddhism, and animist Thai deities. However, the central icon on any Thai altar will always be the image of the Buddha. It is best that the central Buddha icon belong to the Theravada tradition as opposed to the Mahayana (Tibetan or Chinese Buddhism). Other items which may

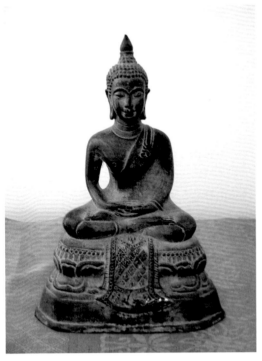

Theravada statue, Thailand. Notice the crossed legs, folded hands, simple clothing, serene unadorned face, and flame headdress.

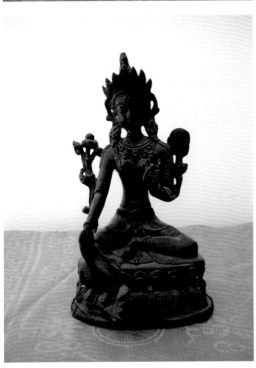

Mahayana Statue, Nepal. Notice elaborate headdress, jewels, legs not crossed, female gender. (This is a statue of a Tibetan goddess.)

be placed on the altar include incense, incense burners, candles, offerings, flowers, vases, and decorative items.

When searching for the perfect icon, keep in mind the fact that Theravada Buddhas may be difficult to find as they are typically made only in Sri Lanka, Thailand, Burma, Laos, and Cambodia, or in larger Western cities with large Southeast Asian populations.

Theravada icons are simple. The lines of the figures are smooth, the robes are plain, and the Buddha's countenance is serene. The Buddha may be shown with an *ushnisha* (cranial bump), a flame, a halo, or a mandorla rising from his top-knot, symbolizing enlightenment, but he will never be crowned or adorned with any jewelry. (See some examples on the next pages, or refer to the many Buddha images throughout this book.)

Westerners are usually more familiar with Tibetan, Chinese, and other Mahayana Buddhist icons. These come from a very different Buddhist tradition and should only be used on a Thai altar as subsidiary icons (as opposed to the central one). Mahayana images may be shown with wrathful faces, elaborate ornamentation, animal heads, or even Tantric sexual imagery. These icons often represent gods and goddesses which are worshipped by the devout, and reflect a much later form of Buddhism heavily influenced by Hindu practices. Another common Mahayana Buddha from China is the so-called "Happy Buddha," a rather overweight individual who is always shown with a big happy smile. This statue represents an incarnation of Maitreya, the Buddha of the Future.

The Theravada Buddha icon is totally different from these examples. As opposed to a depiction of a deity, it is an image of a historical person (Siddhatta Gotama). Thus, the Theravada Buddha is not actually worshipped, but rather is recognized and honored as a great human teacher. The icon is symbolic of the universal principles of wisdom and compassion, insight and love, as embodied in his teachings. When gifts are placed before the Theravada icon, or when Thai Buddhists bow to this icon, it is not so much an act of worship as a symbolic internal gesture which acknowledges these higher

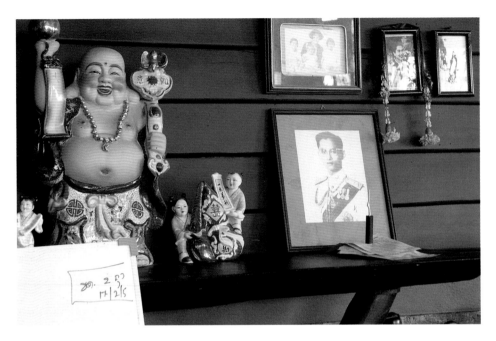

An altar with the Chinese Buddha of the future along with other devotional items, including images of the king and royal family. (Koh Samui)

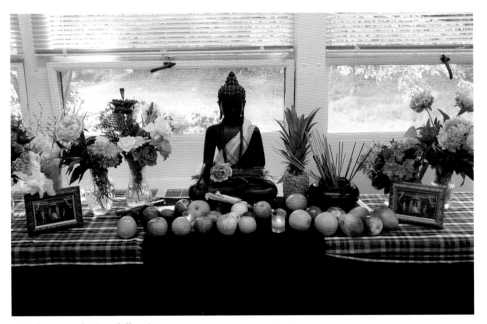

A Theravada Buddha icon.

truths which lie within each of us, and our desire to embody these truths in our lives.

Setting Up a Thai Altar

Centrality and Depth: The altar is a visual expression of hierarchy, and is symbolic of the belief that the spiritual is more important than the secular. The more centrally located an object is, the more importance it takes on. On a Thai altar, the Buddha (sacred) is always more important than the other objects, therefore, the Buddha is always central. Relative importance is also expressed by depth. The more deeply placed an image is (i.e. the more recessed it is), the more importance it has.

In the diagram below, imagine you are standing facing the altar and looking down from above. The surface of the altar is represented by the rectangle. The most important spot on the altar would therefore

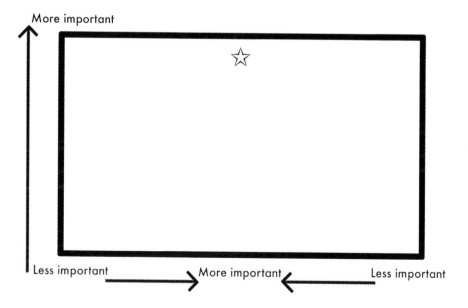

be in the center, farthest away from you (marked by a star). This is where your most important icon should go.

Symmetry: A related concept is the symmetrical layout of the altar. If the most important icon is located centrally, subsidiary images or objects must be placed symmetrically with respect to this. This typically results in configurations of odd numbers of icons, one central image with flanking pairs of subsidiary images (see examples 2 and 4 in next figure). However, layouts can also include even numbers of icons while still preserving the rules of centrality, depth, and symmetry (see examples 1 and 3).

In the examples of altars below, B represents a Buddha and S represents a subsidiary image, either a smaller Buddha, a Jivaka statue, or another type of image. Example 4 below represents the layout of the main shrine at the Traditional Medicine Hospital in Chiang Mai, shown on the following page.

Height: In addition to the above guidelines regarding the placement

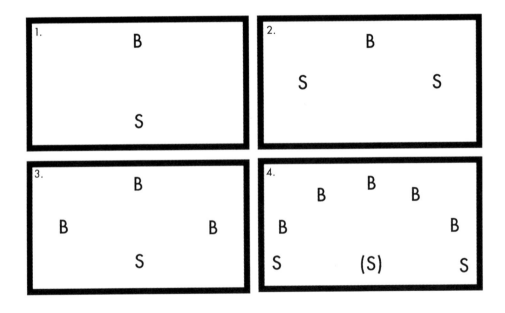

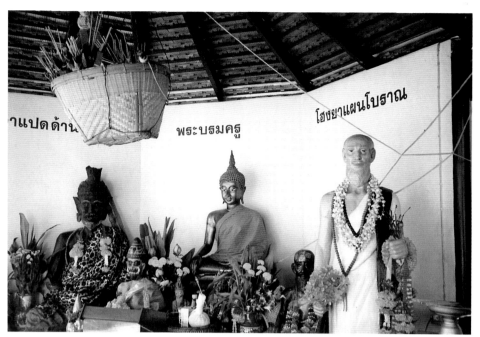

The central altar at the Shivagakomarpaj Traditional Medicine Hospital in Chiang Mai is an example of a traditional Thai Buddhist altar. The Buddha is recessed, central, and flanked by symmetrical subsidiary figures.

of icons, there is one more important consideration: the relative height of the images. The taller the image, the more importance it has. Therefore, your most central image should be tallest, and subsidiary images should be relatively shorter. Keep in mind that a subsidiary image on the left is considered equivalent to a subsidiary image on the right, so they should be approximately the same height.

The examples below are shown three dimensionally, demonstrating 3 inappropriate configurations (a), and 3 solutions to correct these problems (b).

In 1a, the Buddha and subsidiary icon are both the same height. They are both centrally located, and the Buddha is correctly placed

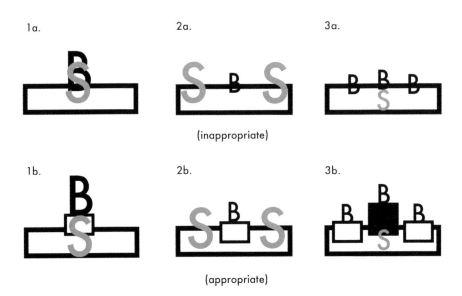

deeper than the subsidiary image. However, in this configuration, the Buddha is blocked by the image in front. The Buddha must be placed higher than the second figure in order to preserve the hierarchy. It is better to raise the Buddha as shown in 1b.

In 2a, the Buddha image is smaller than the other images. Even though it is more central and deeper, the Buddha still must be tallest. This can be corrected again by raising the Buddha image, higher than the subsidiary icons.

In 3a, hierarchy by centrality and depth is OK, but there is no hierarchy by height since all of the images are the same size. Furthermore, the central Buddha is blocked from view by another statue, which is also centrally located. The central Buddha can be raised to correct both of these problems; however, the subsidiary Buddhas must also be raised in order to place them higher than the S, which is not a Buddha, and therefore must be lower.

Offerings: Offerings, such as fresh fruit or sweets, are placed on the altar as gifts to honor the Buddhas and other images. Items such as candles and incense burners should be placed with consideration to

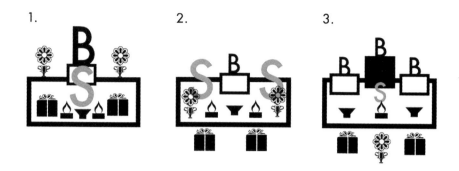

symmetry and height. It is not important how many flower vases, candles, or incense burners you have, only that they are arranged appropriately. These items must not be taller than the icons, must not obscure the icons from sight, and must be placed in such a way as to be visually attractive. Some examples are above:

In altar 1, two flower vases are placed on either side of the Buddha, while 2 candles and a single incense burner are placed directly in front of the subsidiary images. Gifts are placed at the front of the altar on either side.

In altar 2, flower vases are placed on either side of the altar with a central incense burner and 2 candles. Gifts are placed on the ground in front of the altar. (Note that while icons and other sacred images or objects can never be placed on the ground, it is OK to place gifts on the ground.)

In altar 3, a central candle and two incense burners are placed symmetrically on the altar, while gifts and flowers (which are also gifts, and thus can be placed on the ground) are placed in front of the altar. Very tall flowers should always be placed on the ground so as not to be taller than the icons.

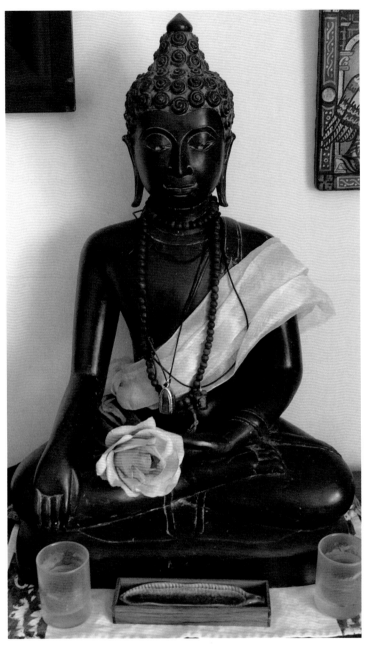

Simple altar layout. Notice symmetrical placement of candles and incense burner. Buddhas can be adorned with certain objects such as beads, icons, and cloth, but it is best to leave the statue as it is unless you know specifically how to decorate it. Other icons can be placed on both sides of (or down in front of) the Buddha.

Setting up a Meditation Space

Room Layout: The altar should be at the front of your meditation area, centrally positioned with respect to the meditation cushions. The cushions should be arranged neatly in rows, or in staggered rows as shown in the diagram below. The order of seating is not important, except for the position of the leader or teacher, who should always sit in the front rightmost seat (marked with a T in the diagram). Leave enough room between the altar and the cushions for the giving of gifts, and enough room between the cushions for participants to approach the altar without difficulty.

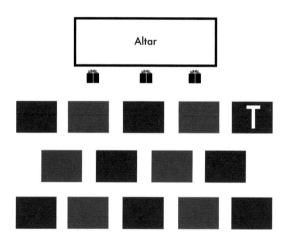

Rules to follow in the meditation space

You should be aware of the following considerations before you use the meditation area for the first time:

• You should remove your shoes (even "indoor shoes" such as slippers) when entering the sacred space.

• You should never point your feet at a Buddha, another image, or any figure (animate or inanimate) deserving of respect. It is therefore only acceptable to sit in the meditation area kneeling (sitting on your heels) or cross-legged.

• You should not point your fingers directly at any of these images either.

- Hats should never be worn.

- You should treat the altar with respect.

- You should not joke, swear, lie, use harsh words, or perform other offensive acts in a room containing a Buddha image.

Exclusivity: This altar is the spiritual focus of the room or house, and it is a sacred space. The altar is therefore not to share space with any secular activity. Supplies should not be stored in the altar's vicinity, nor should food be served. Items not part of the altar should not be placed there. (So don't keep your keys and spare change on it!) Offerings should never be taken off the altar for personal use, such as eating offered fruit. You should also not chat idly around the altar, particularly not when seated on meditation cushions.

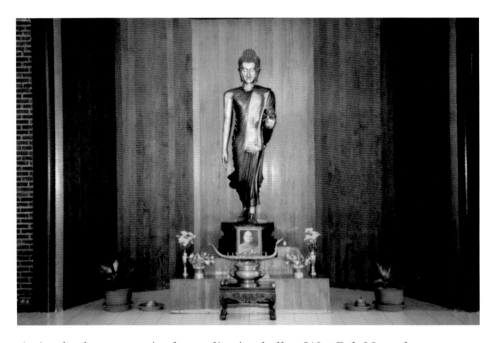

A simple altar set-up in the meditation hall at Wat Pah Nanachat Monastery. (Ubon Rachathani)

Approaching the Altar: With traditional Thai altars, it is important that the icons be placed so that they are located higher than the head of any person in the room. In practice, this sometimes means that smaller altars with shorter icons are placed on shelves on the wall, mounted above head level.

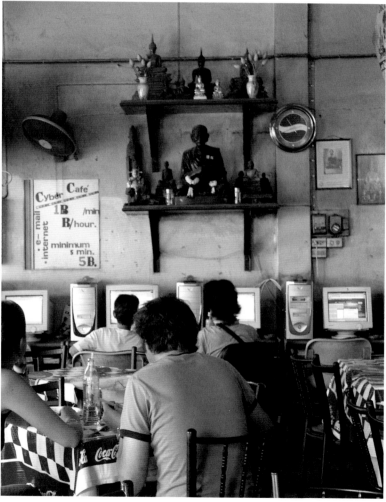

A wall-mounted altar at a Bangkok cyber-café. Traditional Buddhism can be found even in the modern hustle and bustle of the nation's capital. Note the symmetrical layout, and the fact that the Buddhas adorn the top shelf, while figures of monks and other images are kept on the bottom.

However, if this is not possible, you should be aware at all times while in the vicinity of the altar to kneel so as to bring your head down at least to the level of the icons. Shorter icons should not be approached standing, but by first dropping to the appropriate height, and then moving towards the altar. This results in a sort of "shuffling" on the knees which is a signature of respect and honor in Thai culture. This respect is further accentuated by bowing your head to bring it below the level of the icons once you have approached the altar.

Additional Reading

If you are interested in Thai Buddha statues, you may want to consult the following titles:

Standen, Mark and John Hoskin. Buddha in the Landscape: A Sacred Expression of Thailand. Pomegranate, 1999. — This is a fantastic glimpse of the Thai landscape, and the Buddha statues one finds in the most surprising places. Absolutely stunning photos.

Rawson, Philip. The Art of Southeast Asia. Thames & Hudson, 1967. — This book provides an outline of Southeast Asian history and a detailed discussion of the history of Buddhist images in Thailand.

Fisher, Robert E. Buddhist Art and Architecture. Thames & Hudson, 1993. — A broad overview of Buddhist art and iconography, from India to China and Japan. Only a small section on Southeast Asia, but it provides the greater context for the Rawson book.

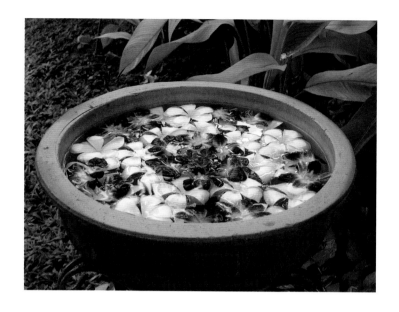

—4—

THE FATHER DOCTOR JIVAKA

Jivaka Komarabhacca

Tradition holds that the founder of Thai medicine is Jivaka Komarabhacca, the personal doctor of the historical Buddha. The earliest Buddhist texts, the Pali canon, mention Jivaka in several places as a wealthy physician and the donor of a mango grove called Jivakarama, which he gave for the use of the Buddha's order of monks as a retreat for the *pansa*, or rainy season.

A detailed biography of Jivaka is provided in the Mahavagga section of the *Vinaya Pitaka*, the monastic "Basket of Discipline" composed in the fourth century BC. In this rather lengthy passage, it is said that Jivaka was an orphan who was raised by a certain Prince Abhaya. When he came of age, he studied medicine with a well-known master in northwestern India, apprenticing with this teacher for a

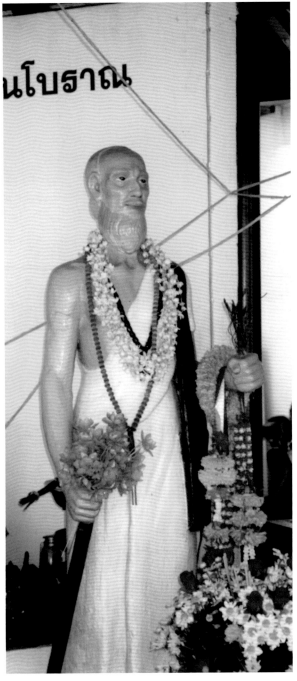

A statue of Jivaka Komarabhacca at the Shivagakomarpaj Traditional Medicine Hospital. Jivaka is always an important figure on the altar of a Thai healer or medical facility, and plays a central role in much of the ceremony surrounding Thai medicine. (Chiang Mai)

period of seven years before returning back home. The biography then tells of six instances where Jivaka healed different individuals, including two instances of major surgery. Among Jivaka's patients were several merchants, the king, and even the Buddha himself, who came to him for a purgative of powdered lotus flowers.

Although the Pali text provides some detail on the practice of medicine in ancient India, historians' knowledge of this period is very sketchy. India at the time of the Buddha was in transition from a strict Vedic system of wrathful war-like gods to more the rational systems of philosophy found in Buddhism and the Upanishads. This also was a period of transition from magical religious medicine based on demonology to the more empirical Ayurvedic medicine.

This transition period lasted many centuries. Ayurveda came into being with the writing of the *Caraka* and *Susruta Samhitas*, two encyclopedic texts which catalogued the medical knowledge of the day. These works were not composed all at once, but both reached their current form by the fifth century AD. When the hatha yoga system was developed in the tenth to thirteenth centuries AD, yoga postures, energy lines *(nadis)*, and pressure points *(marma)* also became part of the medical landscape. These traditions were very influential across South and Southeast Asia, and also form the basis of much of Thai medicine.

Thus, much of the practice of Thai massage and herbal medicine comes from techniques developed in an era 1000 to 1500 years after Jivaka's time. However, there are some similarities with Indian medicine as far back as his era. Therefore, while Thai tradition was by no means fully formed 2500 years ago, Jivaka is revered in Thailand as the founder of Thai medicine.

Many Thais believe that Jivaka developed herbal medicine, Thai massage, and other healing practices himself, and taught these to future generations. The course of history tells us that the transmission cannot be this direct, but it is clear that the roots of much of Thai medicine do lie in the ancient past, and that Jivaka is an important forefather of this lineage.

The *Wai Khru* Ceremony

The *wai khru* ceremony is the most important spiritual practice of the Thai healer, and is a hallmark of Thai medicine. This ceremony is observed at most of the traditional massage and herbal medicine facilities and schools in the country. "Wai khru" (or "wai guru") means "respect the teacher," and this is the formal way in which a teacher or a chain of teachers is honored. The wai khru involves the giving of gifts and a chant by which the practitioners show their debt of gratitude to the lineage of teachers who handed ancient medical knowledge down to the present day. This ceremony centers around Jivaka, but images of more recent teachers may also be included on the altar (in practice, these are always teachers who have passed away).

It is interesting to note that not only traditional medicine practitioners, but shamans, fortune tellers, Thai boxers (muay Thai), tattoo artists specializing in *yan* (see next chapter), and practitioners of many other arts each have their own wai khru ceremonies to pay homage to their own gurus or teachers. Clearly this is a ritual that pervades traditional Thai society.

The wai khru presented here is based on that used at the Shivagakomarpaj Traditional Medicine Hospital to pay homage to Jivaka as the founder of medical tradition. Jivaka is said to descend through the visualizations of the practitioner, in order to bring healing to patients and protection to therapists. The hospital teaches therapists to see themselves as "empty vessels," conduits for the higher powers invoked in the wai khru ritual. The therapist is thus never personally credited with healing powers, and remains humble even with the most spectacular successes.

The idea of Jivaka working through your hands is one that on the surface is difficult for most Westerners to accept literally. However, it also makes sense on the metaphorical or symbolic level. Think of it like this: you are essentially asking for whatever beneficial energies of the universe may be out there to come thorough your hands to help heal the one whom you touch.

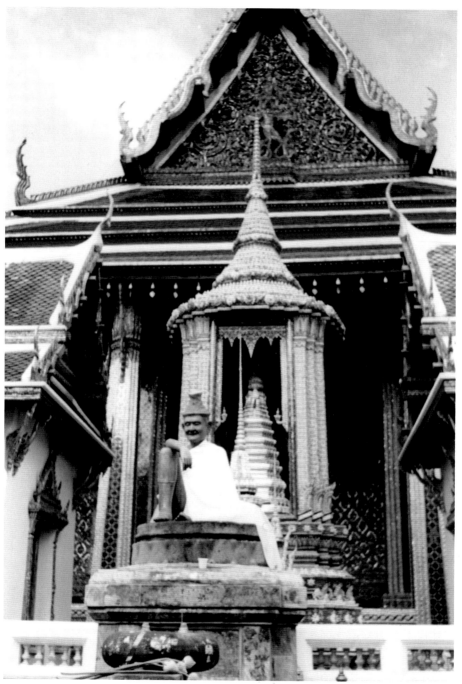

Jivaka presides over the entrance to Wat Phra Kaew. Notice the gold leaf which has been applied to the pedestal by the faithful, and the offering of lotus flowers.

The wai khru ceremony in Thailand is always understood in very devoutly Buddhist way, and you will note that Buddhist language and imagery plays a central role. However, I believe that you need not be Buddhist to participate in or to lead this ceremony. Whether you invoke the Father Doctor or any other positive energy (however this may be personified for you) is not important, I think, so long as the language and performance of the ritual helps to create an intention to tap into this energy for healing purposes. (I will suggest some modifications below for those who are not practicing Buddhists.)

Performing the Jivaka Wai Khru

Once you have set up the altar according to the considerations in the previous chapter, it can be used for the wai khru in honor of Jivaka.

Take a seat on the meditation cushions to begin. From this point, there should be no personal conversations, no food or drink, and no moving around the room. Approach the altar as described in the previous chapter and light the candles to officially begin the ceremony.

Beginning the Ceremony: The traditional Thai ceremony is begun by bowing three times for the Three Jewels of Buddhism: the Buddha, the *Dhamma* (his teaching), and the *Sangha* (the monastic order he founded). This is followed by the repetition three times of the following blessing: *Namo tassa baghavato arahato samma sambuddhassa.* This chant literally means "Homage to the Blessed, Noble and Perfectly Enlightened One."[1]

This triple bow and utterance technically are proclamations of your faith in Buddhism, and therefore, you should not feel that you have to begin your ceremony in this way. On the contrary, unless you are a practicing Buddhist, it is best that you not use this gesture or phrase. (This would be something like a non-Christian performing the Lord's Prayer: it would seem inappropriate to the believers of this religious tradition.)

The alternative way to begin this ceremony is for you to clasp your hands together in the wai gesture (also known as the *namaste* or

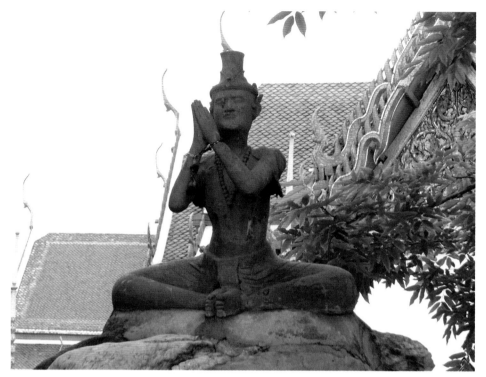

Jivaka giving a "wai" to the faithful at the Wat Pho temple in Bangkok.

prayer gesture), and to bow your head in respect to Jivaka and to the Buddha. Your head should be slightly lowered, not touching the floor as in a full prostration. When paying repects like this, remember that the Buddha and Jivaka statues do not represent deities, but rather human teachers. Or if you prefer, you can think of them as symbolic of the universal qualities of compassion and wisdom.

Om Namo: The heart of the wai khru ceremony is the chant popularly known as the "Om Namo." This chant is performed with hands clasped in the wai. Your head should be bowed, eyes downcast and straight in front of you or closed. Take a deep breath and relax your mind before you begin the chant. You should repeat the following Pali words very slowly, gradually speeding up as they become more familiar.

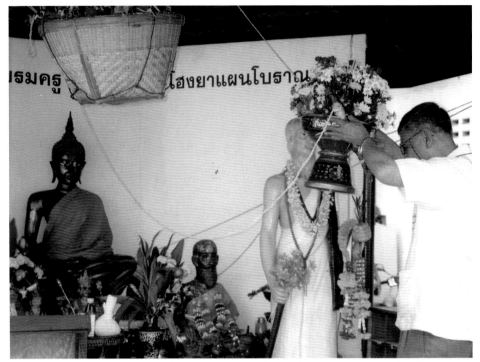

Ajahn Sintorn, director of the Traditional Medicine Hospital, leads the daily wai khru ceremony. (Chiang Mai)

Original Pali text:

> *Om Namo Shivago Sirasa Ahang Karuniko Sapasatanang Osata Tipamantang Papaso Suriyajantang Komarapato Pagasesi Wantami Bandito Sumetaso A-Loka Sumanahomi*

> *Piyo-Tewa Manusanang Piyo-Proma Namutamo Piyo-Naka Supananang Pinisriyong Namamihang Namoputaya Navon-Navean Nasatit-Nasatean A-Himama Navean-Nave Napitang-Vean Naveanmahako A-Himama Piyongmama Namoputaya*

> *Na-ANava Loka Payati Winasanti*[2]

The English translation can be chanted more quickly, at normal reading speed. You can choose from several options...

Prayer by Chongkol Setthakorn:

> *We invite the spirit of our founder, the Father Doctor Jivaka, who taught us through his saintly life. Please bring to us knowledge of nature, and show us the true medicine in the universe. Through this prayer, we request your help, that through our hands, you will bring wholeness and health to the body of our client. The god of healing dwells in the heavens high while mankind remains in the world below. In the name of the founder, may the heavens be reflected in the earth, so that this healing medicine may encircle the world. We pray for the one whom we touch, that they will be happy and that any illness will be released from them.*[3]

Prayer by Ananda Apfelbaum:

> *Homage to you, [Jivaka], who established the rules and precepts. I pray that kindness, wealth, medicine – everything comes to you. I pray to you who brings light to everyone just as the sun and moon do, who has perfect wisdom and who knows everything. We honor you who are without defilement, who are near to Enlightenment, having entered the stream three times. We come to honor you. Honor to you. Honor to the Buddha. I pray that with your help all sickness and disease will be released from those whom I touch.*[4]

These English prayers are not accurate translations of the meaning of the Om Namo. However, I like them. The first is the one used at the Traditional Medicine Hospital, as it is in keeping with the cultural expectations and comfort-zone of most Western students. The second is a bit closer to the actual literal translation, but is still not too overtly Buddhist. The actual literal translation of the Pali is as follows:

> *Homage to you Jivaka, I bow down. You are kind to all beings and bring to all beings divine medicine, and you shine light*

like the sun and moon. I worship he who releases sickness, wise and enlightened Komarabhacca. May I be healthy and happy. He is beneficent to gods and human beings, beneficent to Brahma. I pay homage to the great one. He is beneficent to naga and supanna... I pay homage. Homage to the Buddha... Honor to the Buddha. May all diseases be released.[5]

In this prayer, Jivaka is said to be beneficent to gods and humans, to Brahma (the highest *thewada* or god), and *nagas* and *supannas* (mythical earth-creatures). The meaning is clearly that Jivaka is a universal embodiment of metta, ready to come to the aid of any and all beings in the universe, high or low, near or far. The aim of the Thai healer is to emulate this mission.

Giving of Offerings: Once this chant is finished, gifts are placed on the altar to pay homage to the Buddha and Jivaka. The standard gift is three sticks of incense, although you may present other items as well. The three sticks of incense represent your prayers for well-being, peace, harmony, etc., and again recall the Three Jewels. When the sticks are burned, the smoke rising to the sky symbolizes your prayers rising to the heavens.

Whatever your gift, approach the central area of the altar by moving forward on your knees. Place your gifts on the altar while kneeling, and bow your head in respect while gesturing with the wai. Return back to your seat without turning your back on the altar.

Meditation (optional): Make yourself comfortable while keeping your feet pointed behind you or in crossed-legged position. With eyes closed, practice the meditations from Chapter 2.

Finishing the ceremony: The finishing chant to conclude the wai khru is as follows. Original Pali text:

Araham samma sambuddho bhagava,
buddham bhagavanta abivademi.
Svakkhato bhagavata dhammo,
dhammam namassami.

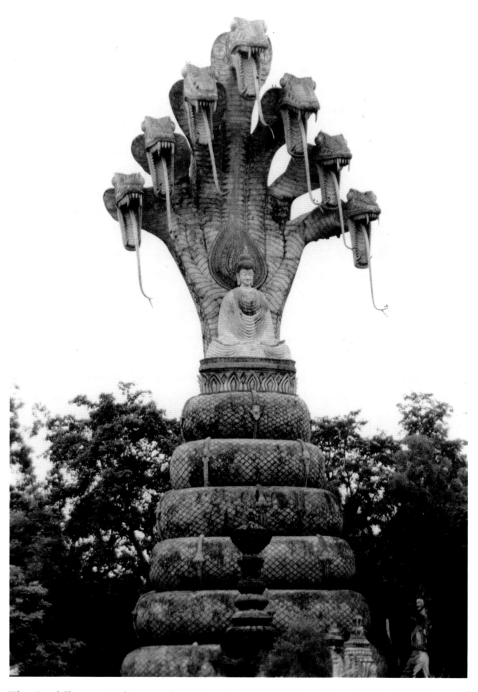

The Buddha, seated in meditation, is shielded from the rain by the king of the nagas *(earth-dragons or earth-serpents) in a popular story from the Pali texts. (Wat Khaek, Nong Khai)*

Supatipanno bhagavato savagasangho,
sangham namami.

English translation:

"The Lord, the Perfectly Enlightened and Blessed One –
I render homage to the Buddha, the Blessed One.
The Teaching so completely explained by him –
I bow to the Dhamma.
The Blessed One's disciples who have practised well –
I bow to the Sangha."[6]

Since this last bit is also a proclamation of faith in the Three Jewels of Buddhism, it should therefore be reserved for practicing Buddhists only. In order to finish the ceremony without this phrase, you can clasp your hands together in the wai, and bow your head in a gesture of respect.

Finally, quietly stand and retreat from the meditation area signifying that the ceremony has ended.

End Notes

1. *Saddhatissa, Ven. Dr. and Maurice Walshe. Chanting Book: Morning and Evening Puja and Reflections. Hertfordshire (UK): Amaravati Publications, 1994,* p. 3.

2. *Chaichakan Sintorn. Traditional Medicine Hospital Handbook for Course in Thai Medicine. Chiang Mai, 1997,* frontispiece.

3. *Chaichakan*, frontispiece

4. *Apfelbaum, Ananda. Thai Massage: Sacred Bodywork. New York: Avery, 2004,* p. 25-26.

5. Trans. by Wijitha Bandara, a Pali scholar at the University of Virginia, in a personal communication, 2005.

6. *Saddhatissa and Walshe,* p. 3.

Additional Reading

If you are interested in the topics discussed in this chapter, you may want to consult the following titles:

Horner, I.B. The Book of the Discipline (Vinaya-Pitaka) Vols. I-VI. Oxford: Pali Text Society, 2000. — The original account of Jivaka's biography and his healing episodes figures in chapter 8 of the Mahavagga section.

Feuerstein, Georg. The Yoga Tradition: Its History, Literature, Philosophy, and Practice. Hohm Press, 2001. — One of the best overall introductions to the yoga tradition. Includes discussions of history, philosophy, and practice.

Wujastyk, Dominik. The Roots of Ayurveda. London: Penguin Books, 2003. — This is a new translation of passages from the most important Ayurvedic texts, including sections of the *Caraka* and *Susruta*.

Zysk, Kenneth G. Asceticism and Healing in Ancient India: Medicine in the Buddhist Monastery. Delhi: Motilal Banarsidass, 1998. — This is a very readable academic book by the foremost researcher of early Buddhist medicine. Zysk discusses the transition from Vedic to Ayurvedic medicine in this short title, and includes a lot of information on Jivaka.

Salguero, C. Pierce. Traditional Thai Medicine: Buddhism, Animism, Ayurveda. Tao Mountain, 2005. — My own contribution to the history of Thai medicine, tracing its origins in Vedic India, early Buddhist tradition, and indigeneous Thai culture.

C. Pierce Salguero

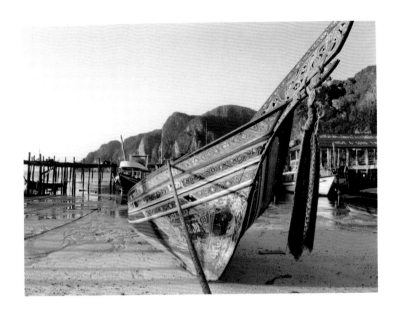

—5—

THE THAI SPIRIT WORLD

Researchers believe that the Thai people originated in Southeastern China or the northern coast of Vietnam. At some point in the latter part of the first millennium AD, the Thais began to migrate out of this region and came to occupy the territory they do today. This ethnic group settled in a region stretching from Northeastern India (Assam) to Laos, and even in parts of Yunnan Province in China. Throughout this vast expanse, there are people who today go by the name Thai, Tai, or Dai, and these people are all from common ancestry.

The people settling in modern day Thailand established the kingdoms of Siam. Most importantly, these were Sukhodaya and Ayudhya, which flourished from the 13th century to the 18th. It was at this time that the Thais came into contact with Indian influence, and that they developed the culture we know today.

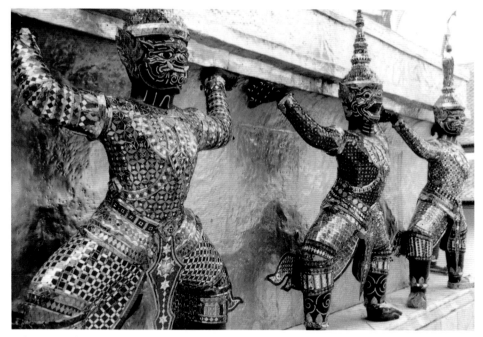

Above: Yakshas *stand guard against any demons trying to enter the temple. They are mythological creatures of giant stature and fierce countenance, but they are said to have been subdued by Buddhism, and entered into the service of good. (Wat Phra Kaew, Bangkok)*

Despite the fact that Buddhism has flourished in Thailand for the better part of 800 years, this religious tradition has by no means replaced indigenous Thai beliefs and traditions which pre-date this time. In fact, many Thai people across Southeast Asia share elements of indigenous practice which must have been traditional in their original homeland. Among these common cultural features is a strong belief in spirits and ghosts.

The Buddhist texts mention several types of angels, demons, and spirits, such as *yakshas* and *kinnaris*. While these do not play a central role in Buddhist philosophy, they are popular folk figures found in dance, storytelling, puppetry, and other arts, and can often be seen in statues on temple grounds. These characters are part of the greater

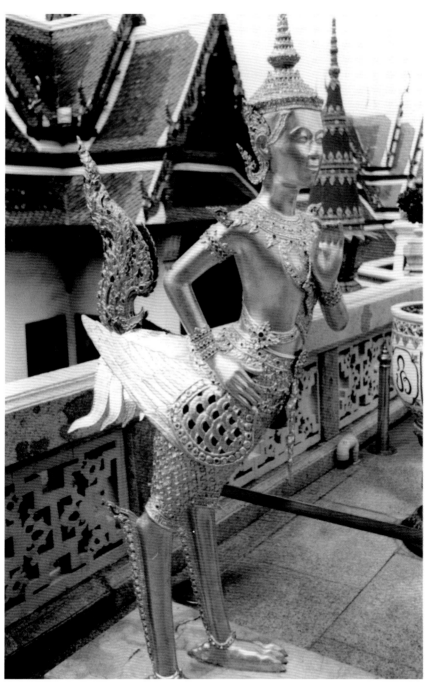

A kinnari, *half woman and half bird, is a figure from popular Buddhist legend who graces many temple grounds. (Wat Phra Kaew, Bangkok)*

Indian heritage, and can be found throughout the Buddhist world.

Additionally, however, the Thai people believe in a large pantheon of spirits with no Indian counterpart. These beliefs relate to the animistic practices of pre-Buddhist times, and exist almost as a separate layer of religion in Thailand today. Animism is the belief that elements of nature are divine. While in the cases below, *khwan* and *phi* are not gods, they are often treated with the respect and fear that deities typically demand, and thus this layer of culture is often referred to as Thai animism.

Phi

Chief among the Thai spirits are the phi (pronounced "pee"). Most phi are evil disembodied ghosts that wander around looking for victims. Many Thais believe that people who die unfortunate, sudden, or violent deaths can become phi and seek revenge for their misfortune. It is dangerous to encounter this type of phi, for they are unpredictable and can cause calamity and disease for anyone who crosses paths with them.

Places that are typical homes for phi are to be avoided. These include secluded ponds, graveyards, deep forests, and locations where misfortune or death has occurred. It is believed that phi can attack humans, possess them, and even kill them. In the Thai hierarchy, monks are considered to be more powerful than phi, so one of the ways to control these spirits is for monks to perform chanting ceremonies. Another recourse is for sick or unlucky people to visit a *phi pob*, or an exorcist, when struck by a disease that has no cure or misfortune that has no explanation.

Often, phi are referred to as "hungry ghosts." Many believe that these spirits are constantly starving, and that they can be tamed and subdued by offerings of food. It is common, therefore, to put offerings of food in places where a phi might enter in order keep them from bothering human affairs.

One example of this belief in phi is the spirit-house. One sees the

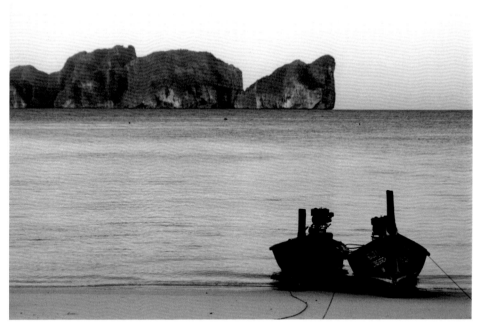

After the 2004 Christmas tsunami devastated the Thai coastline, many Thais abandoned their villages and homes until the phi created by that horrific tragedy could be placated. Only when the temples were rebuilt and the monks returned to the villages did the people move back and begin the reconstruction. (Koh Phi Phi, before being destroyed by the tsunami)

structures all over Thailand in both urban and rural areas. These are small houses built for the earth-phi that is displaced when a new home or other building is built. This is almost like an environmental consciousness personified: it is believed that any time you disturb the land, cut a tree, or build a structure, you can potentially anger a resident phi. Rather than have that phi bothering you and your family for years to come, causing your children to be sick or your business to fail, you should provide the phi with a home of its own that is at least as nice as the one you are building. If these spirit houses are tended daily with offerings of food, water, incense, and other devotional items, the phi will be content and stay away from

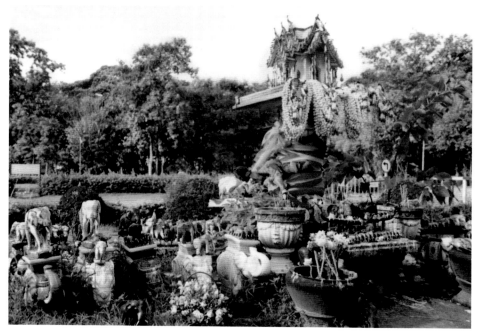

A spirit-house on the grounds of Chiang Mai University is home to the campus phi, and a popular spot for students to give offerings. Note the many elephant statues. These are symbolic of good luck, and are placed at this site by students before exams. Also notice the candles and many sticks of incense from previous offerings.

the human realm. The act of giving of these offerings, known as *wai phi*, is not a means of worshipping the phi, but of keeping it happy. It is a common sight all across Thailand to see people taking care of their phi first thing in the morning, making sure everything is settled in the spirit world before the day's mundane activities begin.

Khwan

Another type of spirit that plays a central role in Thai belief and also in healing is the *khwan*. The khwan is different from a phi because it is located inside you.

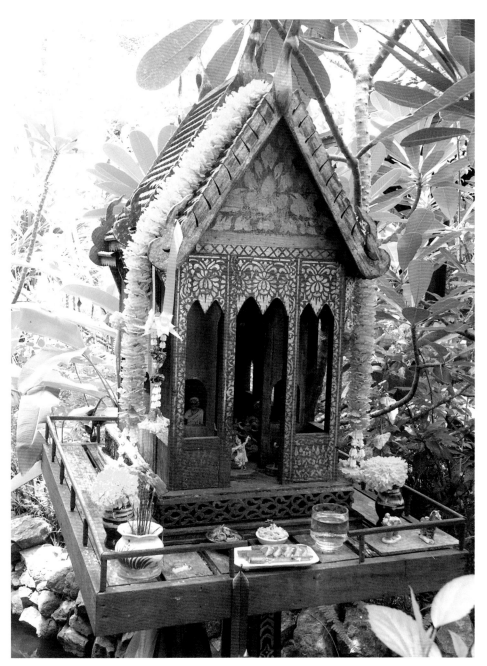

A spirit-house is built as a home for the earth spirit (or phi) which is displaced when a new house or building is constructed on a plot of land. This spirit-house is ornately decorated, to keep the spirit happy and prevent it from inhabiting the human realm. (Koh Samui)

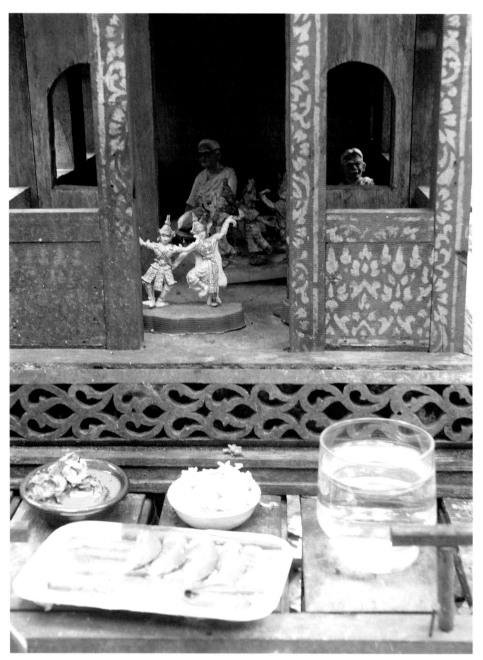

Every day, gifts of fruit, water, rice, curry, flowers, incense, and other items are given to the phi to keep them happy and well-fed. Sometimes spirit homes are furnished, carpeted, and even lit. This house contains small figurines, perhaps symbolizing the phi *themselves.*

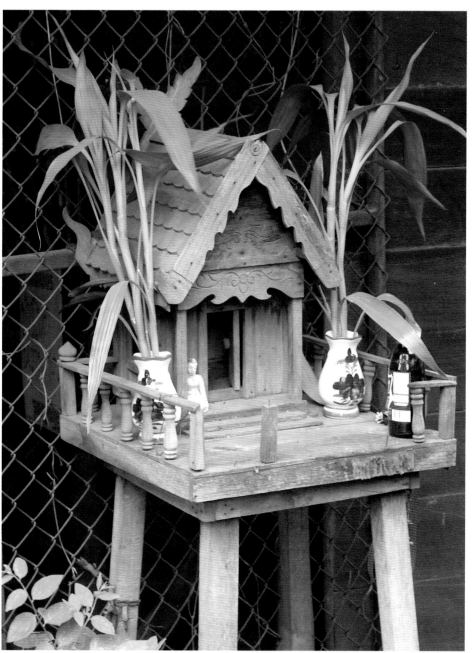

This rural home has a spirit-house that is quite simple. Here, the gifts are not nearly as ornate as in the previous example, but the family still does its best. (Chiang Mai)

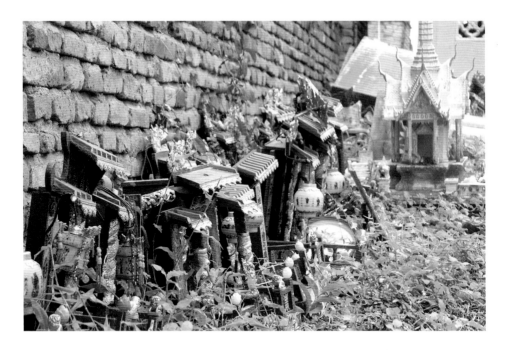

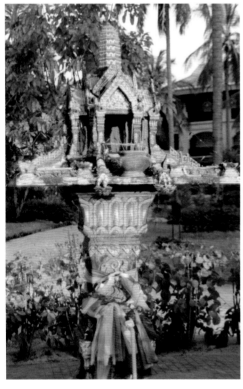

Above: A spirit-house graveyard. When they are falling apart, spirit-houses cannot just be thrown away. They must be deposited in a certain sacred place. This spot is by the city moat in Chiang Mai.

Left: A gilt spirit-house with garlands and other ornate gifts at a resort hotel. (Koh Phi Phi)

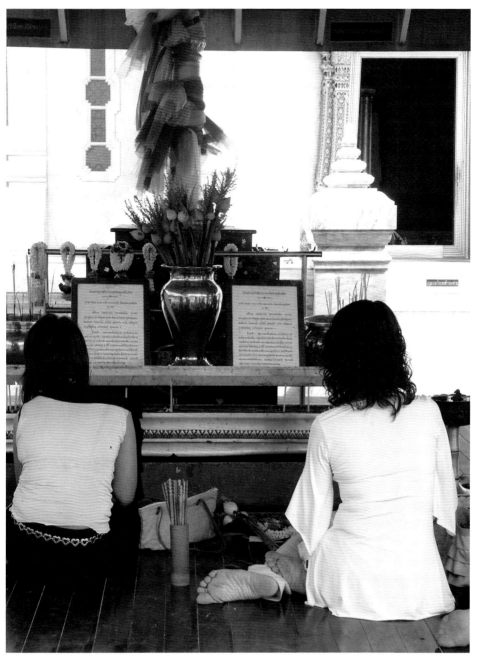

Two women at the Bangkok city pillar. This huge structure (only a part of which is seen in the background) is home to the phi *which guards over the entire nation.*

While the word 'phi' can be translated as spirit, the khwan is more like a soul. We should remember that Buddhism does not believe in an eternal soul that travels from one body to the next in the process of reincarnation. Denial of an external soul is, in fact, one of the distinguishing features of Buddhism that sets it apart from other religions from India—and indeed from around the world. So, the khwan is not necessarily a soul in the Judeo-Christian sense of an immortal piece of you. Rather, the khwan is usually thought of as a "guardian spirit" or as the "essence of life."[1]

As the essence of life, the khwan is a vital part of all living beings, human and otherwise. Some non-human khwan are highly valued in traditional Thai culture. For example, large old trees, particularly Bodhi trees, the species under which the Buddha gained enlightenment (*Ficus religiosa*), are especially revered. These trees often stand on temple grounds because the entire temple structure was built around them. They are often wrapped in sacred cloth, and often their khwan is honored with a spirit-house of its own.

The binding of the tree with sacred cloth is closely related to another Thai custom, the *tham khwan* ceremony. In this practice, the wrists are bound with sacred thread to "tie" the khwan to the body.

It is believed that the khwan can travel outside the body in dreams, and that it can be scared out of the body by a traumatic or frightful event. For example, childhood nightmares and illnesses are often considered to be due to a "lost khwan." Similarly, depression, injury, or mental illness can be attributed to a lost khwan as well. If someone is chronically sick, it may also be due to a wandering khwan. In all these cases, it is believed that the khwan has traveled outside of the body, and cannot find its way back. The tham khwan ceremony can call the khwan back to reunite with the individual, and bind them together to prevent future wandering.

This type of ceremony plays an important role in Thai healing and can be performed whenever someone is sick. As important as any healing technique for the body or energetic system is calling the soul back home, rekindling the essence of life, and getting the individual back to being themselves.

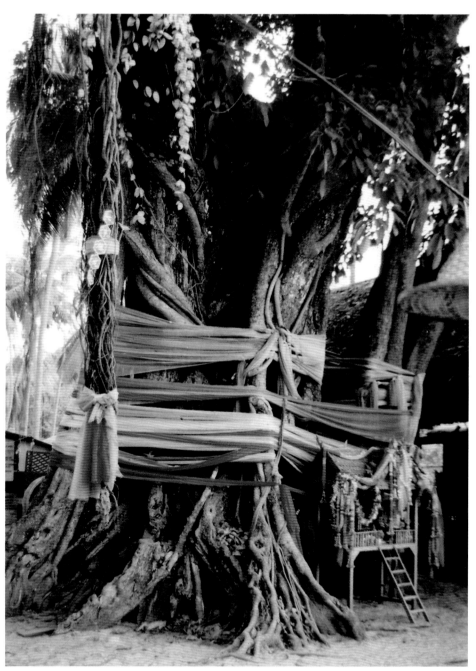

A sacred tree wrapped in colorful cloth to honor its khwan. *Notice the small structure among the roots. This is meant to house the tree's khwan, and also serves as a platform for the presentation of gifts such as food, water, flowers, etc. (Koh Phi Phi)*

Another reason for the tham khwan ceremony is to bind the soul tightly *before* it travels away, to prevent its getting lost. This is frequently done at any kind of "going forth." For example, this can be when a young adult is moving away from the family to start a new life in another part of the country, when a couple is married, when a boy is heading off to become a novice monk, or in any other life transition. In these cases, the family will perform the tham khwan ceremony to bind the khwan and insure the good luck of the one going forth. As they will be far from home and the protection and support of family and friends, they will need to be sure their guardian spirit is with them to watch after them.

The Tham Khwan Ceremony

One tham khwan ceremony I participated in regularly was the graduation ceremony practiced at the Shivagakomarpaj Traditional Medicine Hospital in Chiang Mai. The ceremony begins with the typical chants, and the recitation of the Om Namo phrases from the wai khru in Chapter 4. When this has been completed, the teacher turns to face the students and gives them a word of gratitude for their participation in the training.

The teacher then calls each student forward to receive a diploma, a wai of gratitude specifically directed at them, and their "sacred string." The string is bound around the right wrist to help the individual to maintain a connection with a deeper part of themselves they have been able to access during the course due to the spiritual environment of the traditional hospital. As they go forth into the "real world," their binding string represents a desire for the continuance of this connection between the soul and the self.

This ceremony can be modified to fit any situation. Anyone can bind anyone else's wrist to symbolize the wish for well-being and safety as one heads off into the unknown. As you do so, you can repeat the metta phrases, or something more personal:

"As you go forth from here, may you be happy, may you be well, may you be safe, may you be peaceful, until we meet again."

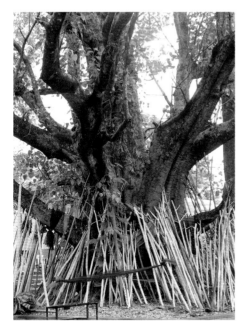 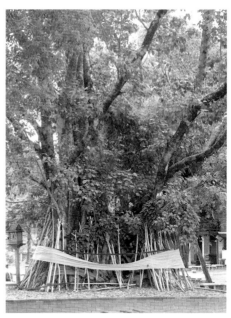

Sacred trees are usually large, imposing, and very old. Many times they are on the grounds of temples, and probably have been growing there for hundreds of years. (Chiang Mai)

If the intent of the tham khwan ceremony is to call a lost soul back home to someone who is ill, troubled, or depressed, the left wrist is bound instead of the right. In this case, the intent is not to bind the soul to the body, but to entice it to come back and reanimate the individual. In this case, the words you choose may be different. You could use the following phrase, or one that resonates with you:

"You have lost your way and are wandering far from here. May you be well, may you be safe, may you be peaceful, and may you find your way home again."

End Notes

1. *Heinze, Ruth-Inge. Tham Khwan: How to Contain the Essence of Life, A Socio-Psychological Comparison of a Thai Custom. Singapore: Singapore University Press, 1982*, p. 17.

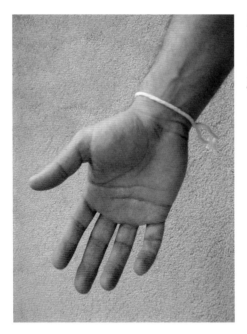

In the tham khwan ceremony, the right wrist is bound with a sacred thread to tie the khwan to the physical body.

Additional Reading

Very little has been written on indigenous Thai spiritual beliefs, but if you are interested in the topics discussed in this chapter, you may want to consult the following academic titles:

Terwiel, B.J. "The Origin of the T'ai Peoples Reconsidered." In Oriens Extremus, 25(1978a):2:239-259. — A detailed discussion of the various theories of the origins of the Thai people and some of the indigenous customs shared by these groups.

Heinze, Ruth-Inge. Trance and Healing in Southeast Asia Today. Bangkok: White Lotus Press, 1997. — Heinze has written many books and articles on spirit-mediums, channels, and possession in Southeast Asia. This book presents case studies of healers, and is a fascinating first-hand account of these types of ceremonies.

Golomb, Louis. An Anthropology of Curing in Multiethnic Thailand. Urbana and Chicago: University of Illinois Press, 1985. – Golomb focuses on exorcism in rural and poor urban Thailand, but this book is a fantastic introduction to the diversity of spiritual healing practice predominant in Southern Thailand.

C. Pierce Salguero

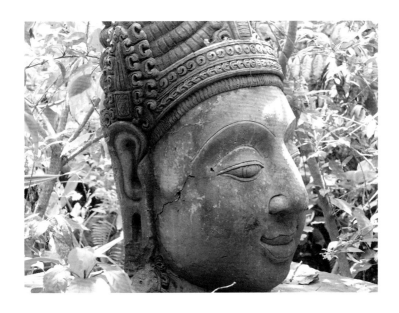

—6—

MYSTICAL SYMBOLISM

Western medicine can be found all over Thailand, and hospitals in Chiang Mai and Bangkok are on a par with those in Europe or America. The first Western hospital was built in the seventeenth century by Jesuits, so these institutions have been around for a long time. However, many Thais feel that the these hospitals only treat the physical body, and seek out other options for treatment of spiritual, mental, and emotional needs. Alongside Western doctors, there are many types of traditional healers in Thailand dealing with these realms. Most are called "mo," or doctors. These include the formally trained *mo boran*, or Ayurvedic doctor, the *mo nuad*, or Thai massage therapist, and the *mo ya*, or herbalist, all of whom study at recognized schools and are licensed by the government.

But the term mo also includes many other unlicensed and unregulated folk-healers who deal with the indigenous spirit world. These include

93

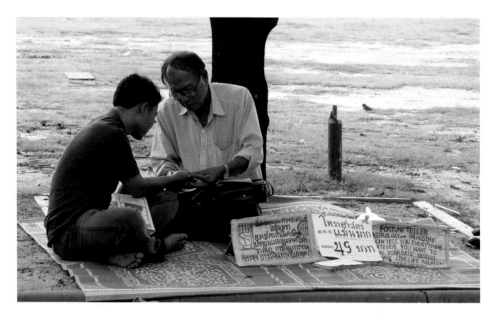

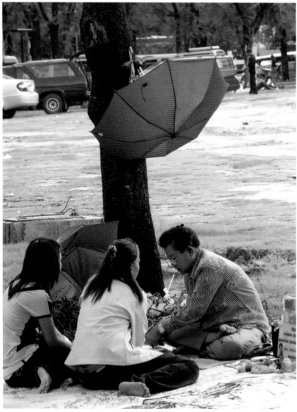

Fortune-tellers and palm-readers frequent the Sanamluang, a central Bangkok park.

the *mo phi pob*, or exorcists mentioned in the previous chapter, and *mo khwan*, specialists in the tham khwan ceremony. There are also *mo phi* (spirit mediums or channels, who become possessed by a spirit which speaks through them), *mo du* (fortune tellers and palm readers who can help divine a person's destiny), and *mo wicha* (those who control magic powers and use these for good or evil), and the list goes on.

Thais are also very passionate about astrology. Ancient texts preserved at Wat Pho (see Chapter 7) mention correlations between health and the day of the week on which someone was born. In popular practice, these indigenous beliefs are blended with Buddhism, and

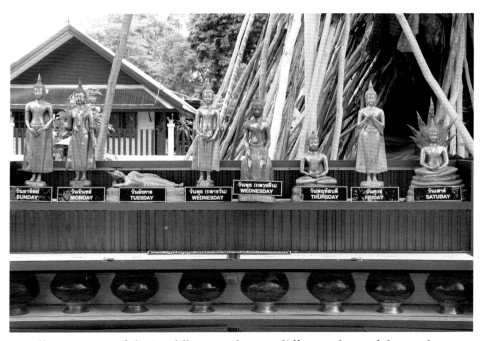

Small statuettes of the Buddha correlate to different days of the week. From left to right are the standing Buddhas for Sunday and Monday, the reclining one for Tuesday, the standing and enthroned ones who both share Wednesday, the meditating one for Thursday, another one in standing posture for Friday, and the naga-sheltered Buddha for Saturday. Alms-bowls placed under each statue are for coins given for good luck by people born on these days.

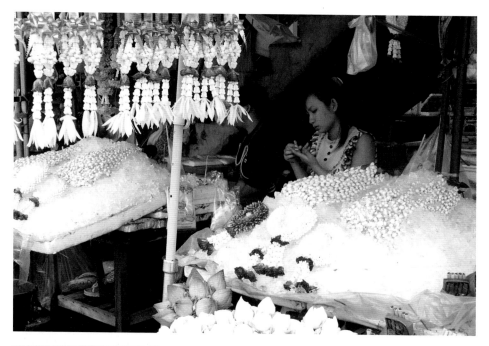

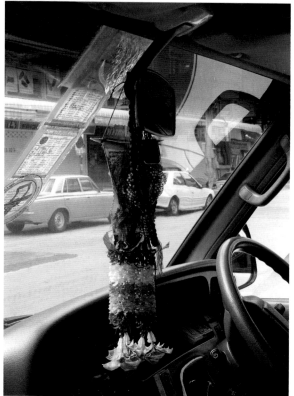

This Chiang Mai girl sells jasmine flower garlands, which are used on rear-view mirrors throughout Thailand to bring the driver good luck and protection. In some areas, this is the only auto insurance available!

many Thais believe that certain Buddha statues bring good luck to individuals born on certain days.

Many modern Thais are quite cosmopolitan and write all of this off as superstition; however, there is a majority of the population that believes in phi, khwan, and mo, and these practices are still extremely popular healing traditions, both in rural villages and urban centers such as Bangkok and Chiang Mai. Many of these folk-healers are women, particularly in the north of the country.

Each of these mo belongs to a distinct lineage, with its own gurus, mythological founders, and wai khru ceremonies. Many mo do not charge for their services, or alternatively they charge a fee based on a pay-what-you-can sliding scale. Usually clients make a small donation to a statue or photo of the mo's guru to make sure the technique is effective.

As described in the previous chapter, consulting a mo is usually the resort of those who have already experienced illness or misfortune. But they can also prevent calamity. In this chapter, I will present the options for warding off phi and other disasters before they strike.

Amulets

One of the chief methods for averting evil and bad luck are amulets. (I am using the word amulet very loosely here, to mean anything which is hung up in a visible place to warn evil forces to stay away.)

One very common type of amulet seen all over Thailand is the jasmine garland. These are strung by hand and sold at stalls in every market. Jasmine garlands are not usually worn, but rather are used to adorn altars, spirit houses, and other locations, or as offerings. Alternatively, they are also hung on rear-view mirrors to ensure luck and safety while on the road.

Another extremely popular type of amulet is a small glass-encased statuette which is worn around the neck on a chain, always in odd numbers. These amulets can be images of a folk-deity or a renowned

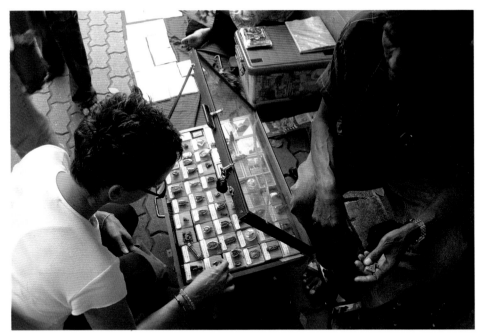

Amulets come in various sizes, shapes, and prices. Some are authentic antiques, and some are cheap plastic imitations. The purchaser must do a lot of research before settling on the perfect one.

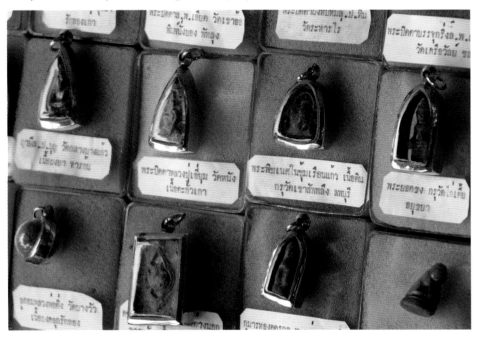

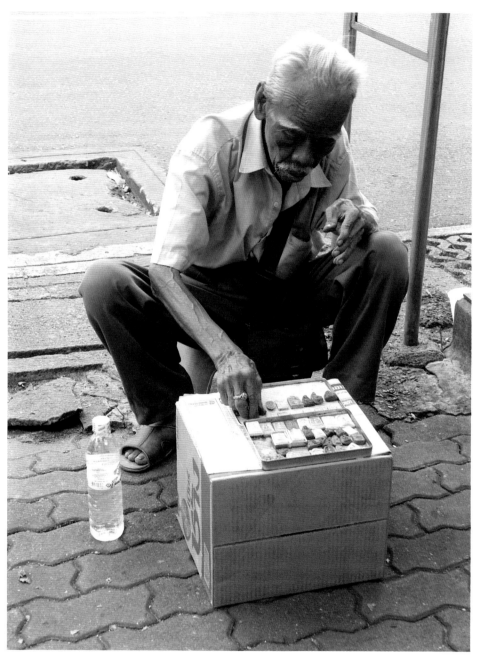

Selling amulets outside of Wat Mahathat, Bangkok.

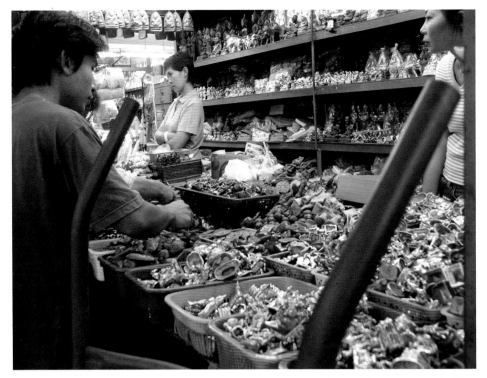

The amulet market has thousands of statuettes to choose from. (Bangkok)

monk who is said to have certain powers. More often, however, these amulets are images of the Buddha.

These days, cheap amulets made from plastic and inexpensive resins can be found in the markets. Typically, however, more powerful amulets are usually made of special ingredients. For example, when a temple is rebuilt, the building materials of the old structure which can not be reused might be pulverized and made into amulets. Similarly, wood from old sacred trees, or fossilized bones, or even ashes from a deceased teacher can all be ground up and mixed with other ingredients to make amulets. Based on the ingredients used and the image carved into it, different amulets have different properties. Some are designed to bring good luck, and others to avert bad luck. Most mo will carry at least one amulet in order to ward off evil influences and to augment their healing powers.

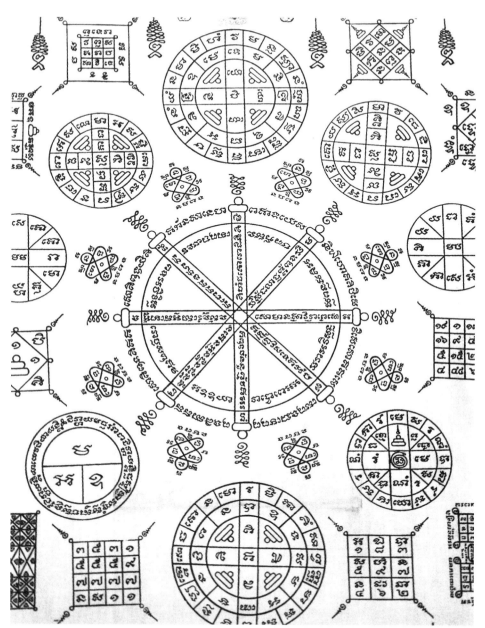

A yan, *or mystical picture, is constructed with magical syllables and symbols. Yan can be painted on walls, the ceilings of cars, or other locations to bring good luck, protection from evil, and health. Many homes and businesses hang a yan above the doorway to attract good luck and money.*

Yan

Many amulets have carved into them a mystical symbol, or *yan*. Yan are also used separately from amulets as they are powerful in their own right. Yan are closely related to a type of art known across Asia. The Tibetan Buddhist tradition uses *yantra* and *mandalas*, both very similar to Thai yan. The Chinese use magical seals in esoteric Taoist healing and religious rituals as well. The Thai yan are also closely related to similar symbols used in Cambodia, Laos, and elsewhere in Southeast Asia.

Thai yan are made up of a wide variety of symbols. The meaning of each yan is different—ranging from bringing luck and money to preventing attack by evil spirits—and are difficult for the outsider to grasp without knowing the detailed symbolism of the tradition. Among those elements used are stylized images of Buddhas and folk-deities, powerful animals like tigers and turtles, and magically potent syllables from Thai, Pali, Sanskrit, and Khmer languages. These elements are combined in geometric designs based on cosmological symbolism and numerology.

A common way of utilizing yan is to have them tattooed onto the body itself. This cross-cultural practice is related to similar traditions found throughout Southeast Asia and Oceania, from the Pacific Islanders of Fiji and Samoa to the Maoris of New Zealand. Across this wide geographical range, tattooing is considered to be a mark of strength, virility, and manhood. (Women are not tattooed in most of these traditions.) Among the Thai 100 years ago, most men were tattooed, many from waist to knees.

Today the tattoos are most popular with members of the military and police forces, as well as others who come into regular contact with danger. This can also include many different types of mo, who consider themselves to be constantly in danger as they deal with unpredictable phi and other malevolent forces on a daily basis. Often, these individuals will wear amulets, consult mo du to determine their lucky and unlucky days, and go through other steps to protect themselves. However, many will also literally cover themselves in

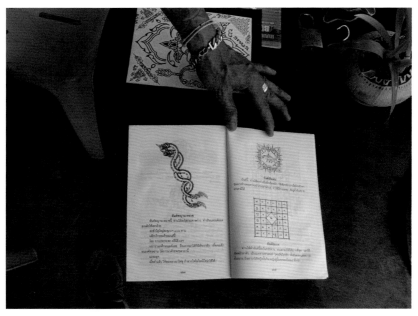

Instruction manuals for tattoo artists, explaining how to draw yan and interpret their meaning.

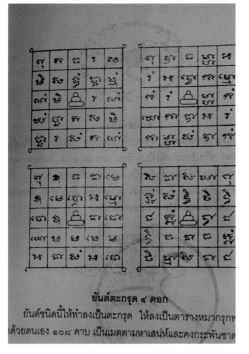

ยันต์ตะกรุด ๔ ดอก
ยันต์ชนิดนี้ให้ทำลงเป็นตะกรุด ให้ลงเป็นตารางหมวกกระทุก
ด้วยตนเอง ๑๐๘ คาบ เป็นเมตตามหาเสน่ห์และคงกระพันชาต

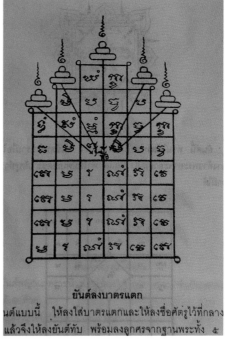

ยันต์ลงบาตรแตก
นต์แบบนี้ ให้ลงใส่บาตรแตกและให้ลงชื่อศัตรูไว้ที่กลาง
แล้วจึงให้ลงยันต์ทับ พร้อมลงลูกศรจากฐานพระทั้ง ๕

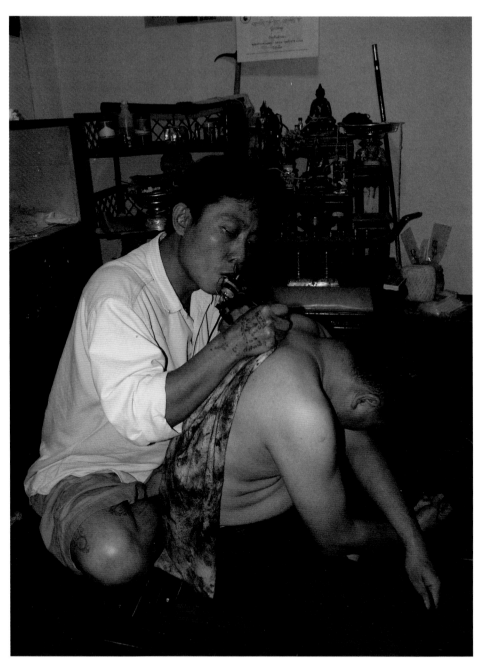

A tattoo artist who specializes in yan. As he works, he chants powerful phrases to empower the tattoo. Notice the altar in the back. In addition to Buddhist icons, this altar includes images of the artist's guru, and each client must pray before the altar when the tattoo is completed. (Chiang Mai)

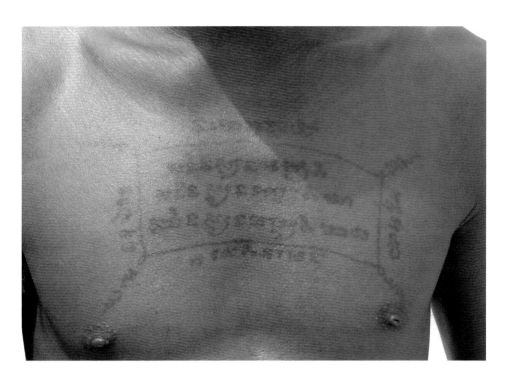

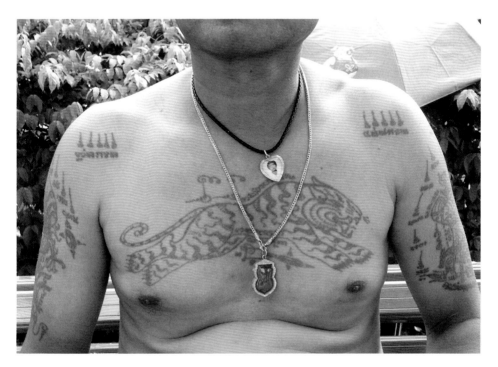

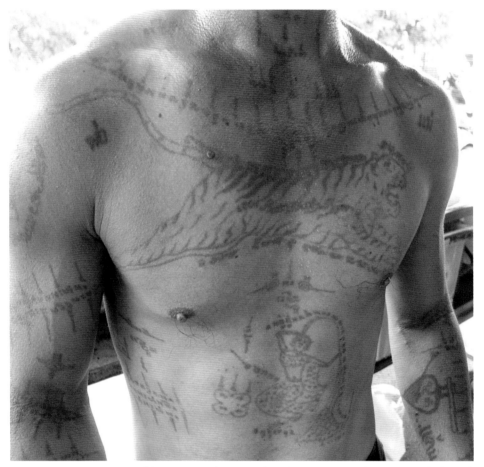

Some men are covered in tattooed yan. The tiger, or Singha, is symbolic of strength and courage.

magical tattoos for added protection.

Tattoos can have a wide range of magical powers. Some are said to bring the wearer increased health, strength, sexual vitality, or good luck. Others are said to make the wearer impervious to bullets, to knife-wounds, and to car accidents.

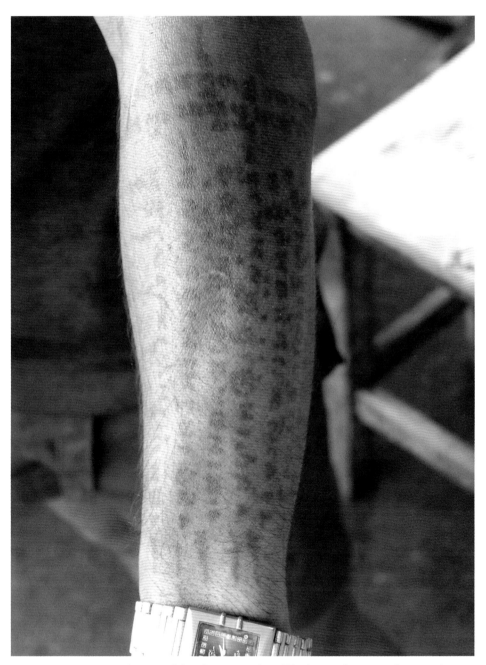

Yan tattoos are written with Khmer script, Thai numbers, and esoteric Buddhist and animist symbols.

Additional Reading

Almost nothing has been written on the topics covered in this chapter outside of narrowly academic circles, but you may find this book interesting:

McCabe, Michael. *Tattoos of Indochina: Magic, Devotion, and Protection – Thailand, Cambodia, Laos. Atglen, PA: Schiffer Publishing Ltd., 2002* – A colorful book by a tattoo aficionado looks at various yan tattoo traditions in Southeast Asia.

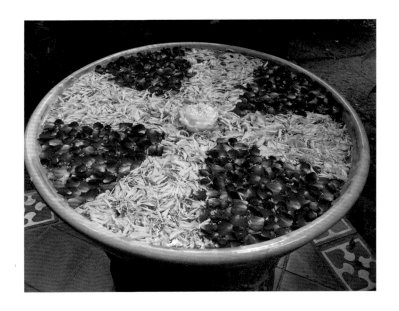

—7—

THE WAT PHO ROYAL TEMPLE

The Thai Temple

Perhaps the most visually interesting example of Thailand's varied cultural influences is the Thai temple or *wat*. Some are quaint simplistic buildings, and some are the most dazzling complexes on Earth, but all are a unique meld of architectural styles, mosaic designs, and devotional art.

All Thai temple complexes are planned out according to ancient Indian Vedic tradition, but the buildings on the grounds are uniquely Thai and feature may of the folk-deities we have already met. Thai temple buildings are topped with characteristically spiked roofs. Each curlicue spire is a meter-long stylized head of an eagle or a serpent, searching the skies to ward off evil spirits. Two massive *nagas*, or serpent-gods, guard the doorways to the wat for the same reason, and typically their elongated bodies serve as rails for the staircases

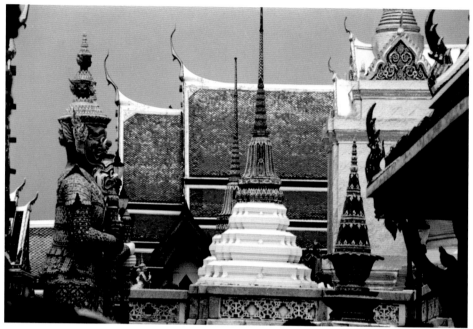

The glittering grounds of Wat Phra Kaew, adjacent to Wat Pho, are among the most striking destinations in Thailand. Note the nagas or eagles on each roof, and the yakshas standing guard.

that lead up to the ornate doors. *Yakshas*, with terrifying faces, stand guard at the gates.

Wats differ depending on the epoch of their construction and the population they are meant to serve, and the interior is as variable as the exterior. Most have high vaulted ceilings and tall narrow windows, but some temples are dark and cathedral-like, while others are airy and bright. Some temples lack walls, to let in a wonderful cross-breeze.

The main hall, or *sala*, usually houses the principal Buddha image of the wat, and is considered the most important building on the grounds. The sala's altar is an explosion of flowers, offerings, and images, figurines of the Buddha and his disciples, statuettes of abbots past and present, busts or portraits of the king, and the main Buddha

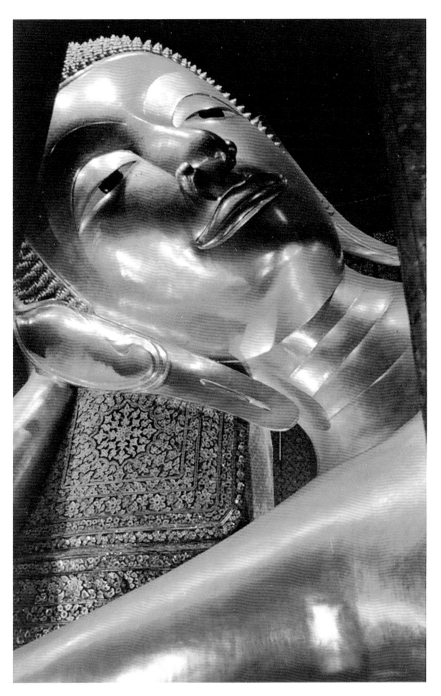

The huge reclining golden Buddha in Wat Pho's sala.

image (this is always a Theravada icon, see chapter 2 for details) — and much of this is covered in gold-leaf applied by the laypeople who come to visit. Once in a while, each statue is cleaned and buffed to turn the flaky leaf into smooth sheets of gold, and thus all of the bronze pieces are slowly converted to glittering gilded reminders of the temple-goers' devotion.

The exterior of a temple building is usually encrusted with intricate mosaics laboriously made from millions of pieces of Chinese porcelain, colored glass, gold leaf, tile, and mirrors, and when this catches the sun, the entire complex sparkles brilliantly. Various other similarly decorated buildings serve as libraries, meeting halls, and classrooms, and the grounds are festooned with colorful *chedis* (or pagodas) housing sacred relics or ashes.

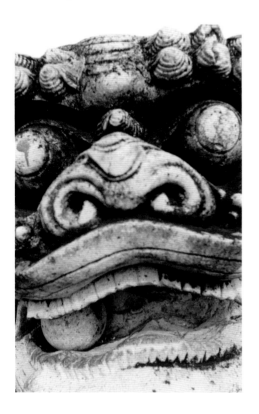

A Chinese-style guardian dog protects a passageway. While there are examples of some Chinese influence in Wat Pho's artistic program, the temple's focus remains on showcasing traditional Thai culture.

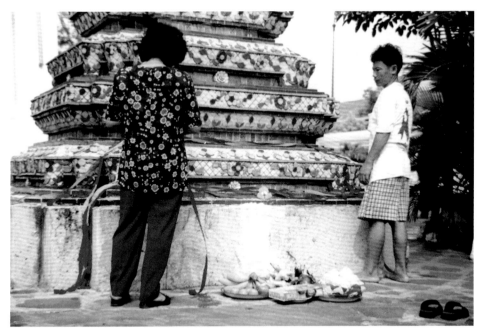

A chedi *on the grounds of Wat Pho. Notice that the surface is encrusted with ornate porcelain tiles. This family is wrapping the chedi in a sacred cloth, and are giving offerings of fruit, flowers, and incense. No doubt this is to honor the person whose ashes are installed within the chedi.*

The Royal Temple of Wat Pho

One of the most impressive temples in Thailand is Wat Pho. The current facility was built in the early 1800s on the site of a monastery that had been active for centuries. The time of the reconstruction coincided with the move of the capital from Ayudhya to Bangkok after a crushing defeat at the hands of the Burmese army. With their old capital in ruins, all art destroyed, the libraries burned, and society in disarray, the new Bangkok dynasty rebuilt Wat Pho as a royal temple intended to initiate the reconstruction of Thai culture itself.

At this time, Wat Pho was designated a repository of Thai cultural heritage, and was opened to the public as a universal educational facility. All of the Thai arts and sciences were showcased and

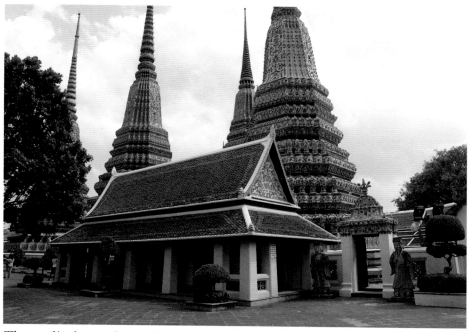

The medical pagoda on the grounds of Wat Pho.

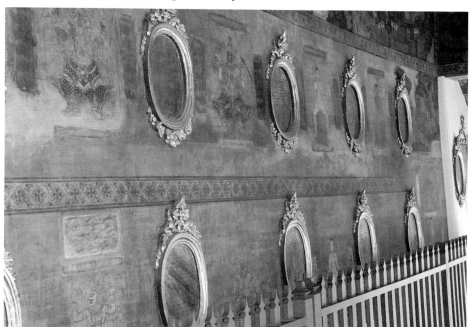

Marble tablets with herbal recipes are mounted in the medical pagoda.

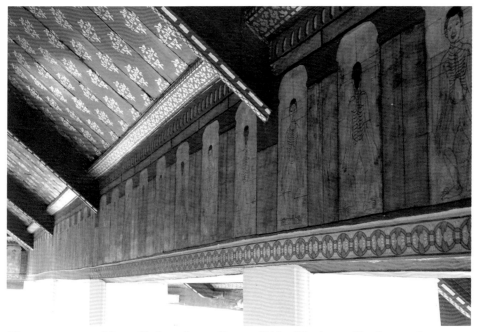

The massage tablets, lining the ceiling of Wat Pho's medical pagoda.

preserved within the temple walls. Various schools of Thai sculpture, bronze-casting, painting, and architecture were preserved, as was Thai knowledge about mathematics and astronomy. Among the sciences thus preserved was traditional Thai medicine. As virtually all of the important Thai medical texts were destroyed in Ayudhya, this project required bringing together medical experts from all over the land to share their expertise, and compiling a definitive version of the lost texts.

In the 1830s, the result of these conferences was the production of tablets which preserved medical knowledge in stone. These tablets were mounted in the medical pagoda on the grounds of Wat Pho, where they can be seen today. Many tablets relate to Thai massage therapy, acupressure, and energy-line theory. Others list herbal recipes. These artifacts form the basis for all of the massage and

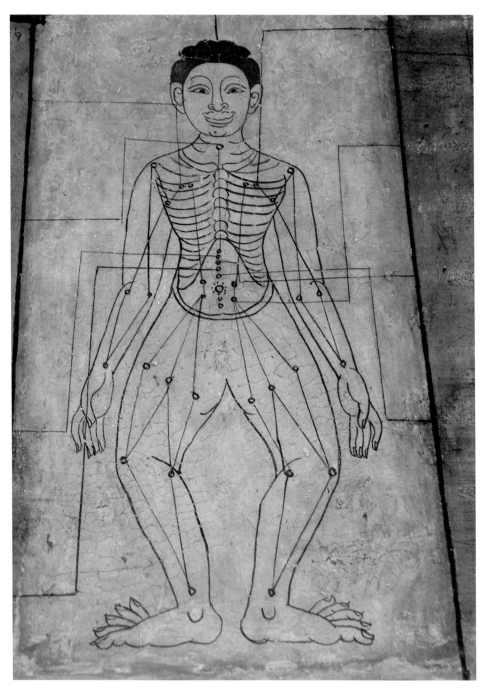

A tablet depicting sen *(energy lines) and* jap sen *(acupressure points) for treatment of diseases and disorders.*

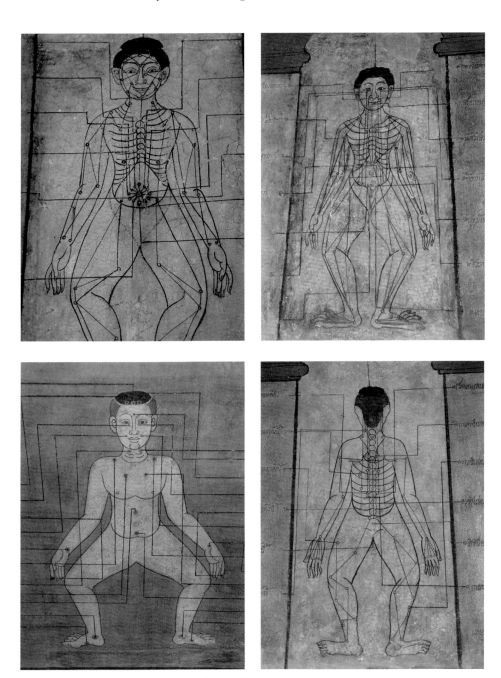

More tablets from the medical pagoda.

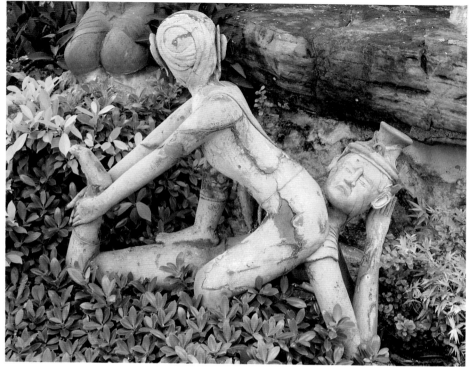

The last remaining statue at Wat Pho depicting massage. The accompanying inscription says this is a cure for testicular hydrocephaly.

herbal licensure programs in the country.

Additionally, a number of statues dating from the same period can be found in small gardens which depict *rishis* (wise men) performing yoga poses and Thai massage steps. Unfortunately, of the 80 statues made, many have been destroyed, and only one remains depicting Thai massage. The remainder demonstrate a type of individually-practiced yoga therapy known as *ruesri dut ton*, in which specific stretches and pressure points are shown for specific ailments.

Although it is no longer a working monastery and has become a tourist attraction, with its grand Buddha statues and ornate salas, Wat Pho remains an active center of Buddhist ritual and practice.

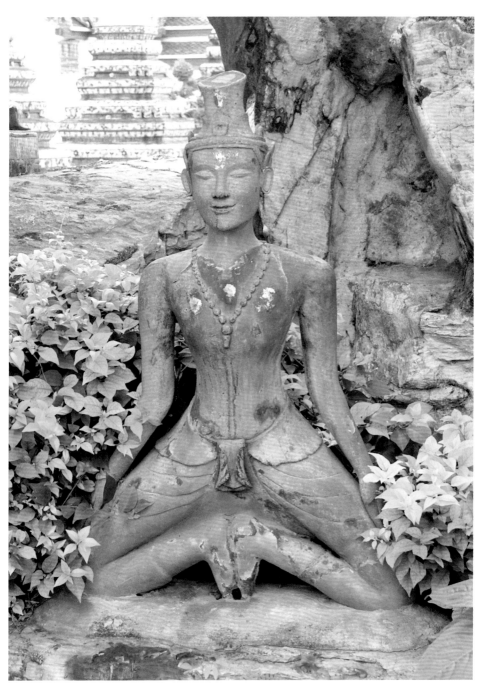

According to the inscription, this rishi *shows a posture to relieve sciatica.*

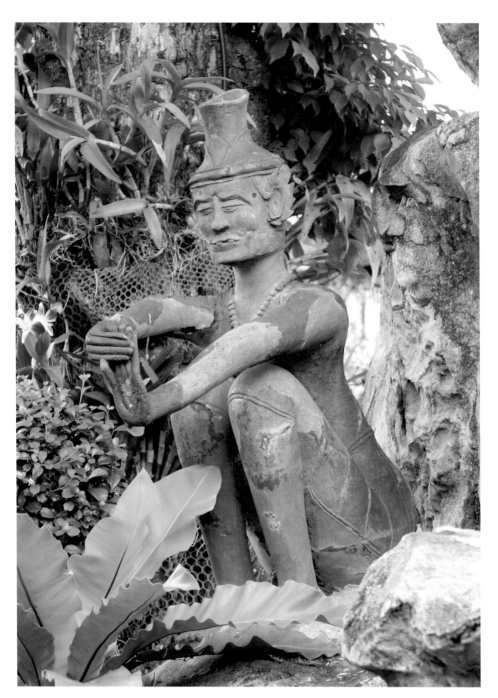

This posture is called the "Four Ascetics Blended Together," a treatment for stiff arms.

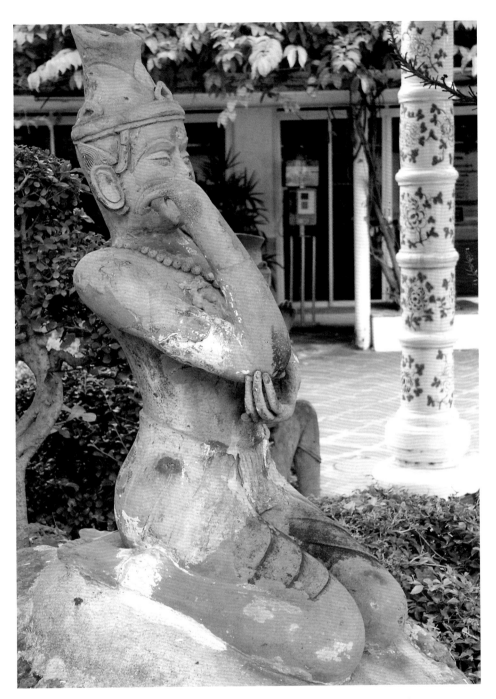

This is the rishi Vyadhipralaya, *demonstrating a posture said to treat stiff hands and feet.*

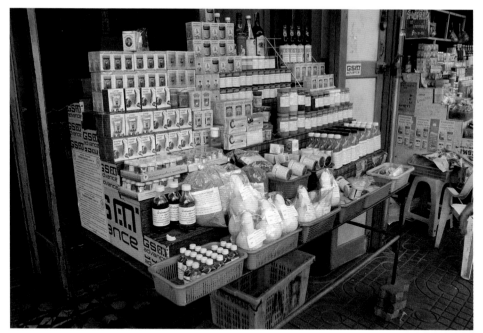

Outside of Wat Pho vendors sell dried medicines, salves, and herbal compresses. Wat Pho is considered to be the top herbal school in the country, although there are many other institutions which offer licensure programs as well.

The fact that this famous university of traditional Thai culture began on the grounds of the royal temple is indicative of the central role monasteries have played in the development of traditional Thai medicine. Up until recently, traditional Thai medicine was often practiced within the grounds of a monastery, or closely connected with a temple.

Wat Pho today still houses a school of Thai massage and herbal medicine, and continues to provide leadership in traditional medicine. In the past ten years, the Wat Pho medical school has been at the front of a national effort to standardize and promote traditional Thai medicine as a viable alternative to Western hospital-based medicine. This project has succeeded in implementing a national licensure program which requires schools and massage clinics to be properly standardized and accredited. However, while this law has improved the quality of Thai medical facilities, it also has threatened the practices of the healers practicing local variations of traditional medicine which do not conform to the national curriculum. Going forward, the future of traditional medicine in Thailand will depend on the interactions between established licensed schools like Wat Pho and those unlicensed traditional healers like the ones discussed in the last two chapters.

Additional Reading

If you are interested in Wat Pho, you may want to consult the following book:

Matics, K.I. A History of Wat Phra Chetuphon and its Buddha Images. Bangkok: Siam Society, 1979. – A photographic tour of the temple, with a short history written by the foremost Western scholar on Wat Pho.

C. Pierce Salguero

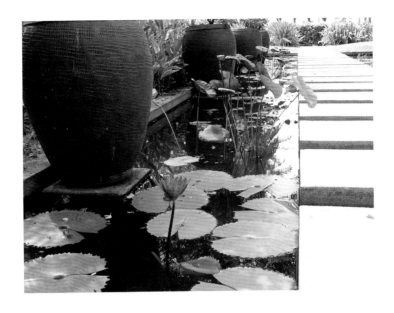

—8—

CHIANG MAI:
CENTER OF TRADITIONAL THAI HEALING

Chiang Mai, nicknamed "The Rose of the North," is the capital of Thailand's northwestern region. This area was for centuries the nation-state of Lanna, a separate entity from the Siamese kingdoms of central Thailand. As the old name four Southeast Asia, Indochina, would suggest, this entire region historically has been at the crossroads between the two great cultures of the Indian subcontinent and imperial China, and nowhere is this more apparent than in Chiang Mai. Erected on the Mae Ping River in 1296, the city historically linked China's Silk Road to Southeast Asia, and long served as a cultural and commercial hub between the Muslim community in southern China's Yunnan region, the Indian kingdoms of Burma, the Khmers in Cambodia, and the Theravada Buddhist people of central Thailand.

Chiang Mai is Thailand's second city, with a huge tourist population, and as such it is modernizing much more quickly than other areas of the country. But despite this inevitability, the city continues to display tangible reminders of its rich multi-cultural heritage. The blocks of teak houses that are quickly disappearing in other Thai cities still seem to be thriving here. Pedestrian alleys paved with brick connect these neighborhoods to community temples and markets, and even staying in a downtown guest house, you can easily imagine you are in a small village instead of a city of well over a quarter of a million people. Chiang Mai is actually a nice blend of both worlds: 700-year-old structures, ancient temples, and quiet neighborhoods coexist alongside modern malls, hospitals, and all of the amenities and conveniences of life in the 21st century — all on a much smaller and more pleasant scale than Bangkok.

One of the most interesting aspects of Chiang Mai is its proximity to the Hill-Tribe regions. Just north of the city, the Golden Triangle is formed by the border between Thailand, Burma and Laos. The area's virgin forested mountains are the first foothills of the vast ranges that culminate in the Tibetan Plateau, many hundreds of miles to the northwest. This area is still as undeveloped as ever. The region's tribal population of roughly 700,000 people includes about 1200 villages belonging to six distinct tribes: the Karen, Hmong, Lahu, Akha, Lisu, Yao, and Lawa, all of which are related to the Tibetan people of the Himalayan highlands. In addition, there are large numbers of Burmese living in the mountain settlements, refugees fleeing the oppressive military government of Myanmar.

Most of the tribal villages still retain their traditional culture and gain their livelihood by wet-rice cultivation. In addition, Hill-Tribe families raise pigs and practice subsistence vegetable farming, and supplement their income with whatever cash they receive from marketing their handicrafts and other wares in Chiang Mai. Hill-Tribe artwork can be seen everywhere on the streets of the city. Hill-Tribe merchants in the Night Bazaar, catering to Thais and tourists alike, offer embroidery, batiks, silver jewelry, teak carvings, lacquerware, woven baskets, and antiques for sale.

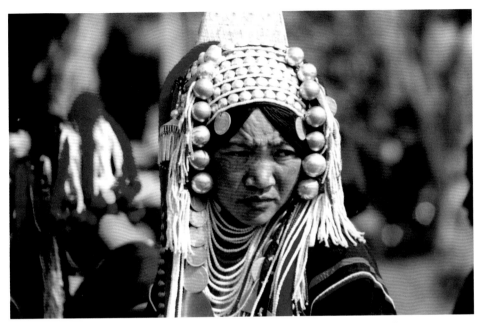

The Chiang Mai area is home to Hill-Tribe people, many of whom continue to observe traditional customs of dress and arts, demonstrating their beautiful silversmithing and loom-work.

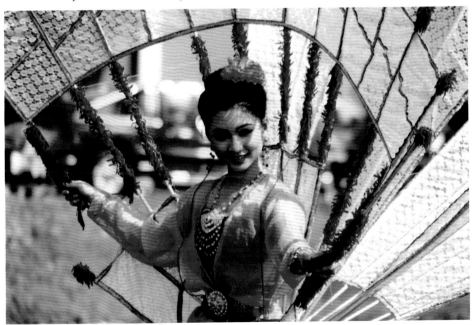

A peacock dancer poses during the annual Flower Festival, a celebration of traditional Lanna culture.

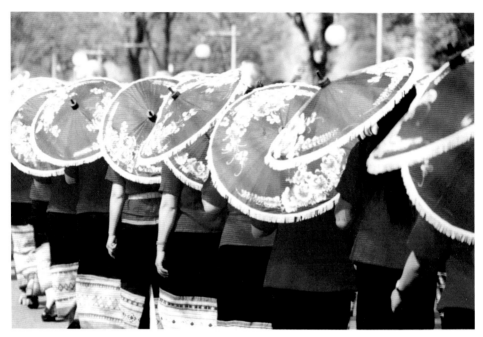

More scenes from the Chiang Mai Flower Festival.

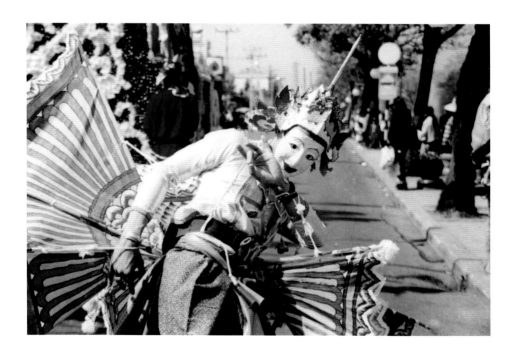

In addition to the indigenous Hill-Tribe culture, other forces are at play in this colorful city. A large Chinese minority inhabits Chiang Mai (as in most other Thai cities) and the influence of this affluent group stretches to all areas of life. Almost everywhere—from storefronts to menus to product labels—one can see Chinese characters side by side with the Thai script.

The section of Chiang Mai consisting of predominantly Chinese businesses (known of course as Chinatown) is a thriving commercial district. This area, complete with flashing neon signs, Chinese-speaking proprietors, and late-night noodle shops, could be any Chinatown in the world. Situated along the west bank of the Mae Ping River, this area is one of the most colorful parts of the city and a thriving center for medicinal herbs.

Outside of Chinatown's huge Warorot Market, traditional Thai pharmacies offer an assortment of aromatic powders, herbal compresses, dried herbs, and pickled insects, which are popular panaceas for a whole range of ailments.

The Shivagakomarpaj Traditional Medicine Hospital

Chiang Mai is a center for the study and practice of traditional medicine of all types. There are Ayurvedic doctors, Chinese medical schools, and more Thai massage clinics per square kilometer than anywhere else in the country. Among these, the Shivagakomarpaj Traditional Medicine Hospital ranks as the foremost.

This facility, commonly known by its nickname "Old Medicine Hospital," is one of the most prestigious traditional medicine centers in Thailand, and was the first in Chiang Mai to open its doors to Western tourists wishing to learn Thai massage. Their 10-day course continues to be the best introductory class in Thai massage around. For those who speak Thai fluently, the hospital offers formal training programs in traditional Thai medicine which result in national licensure.

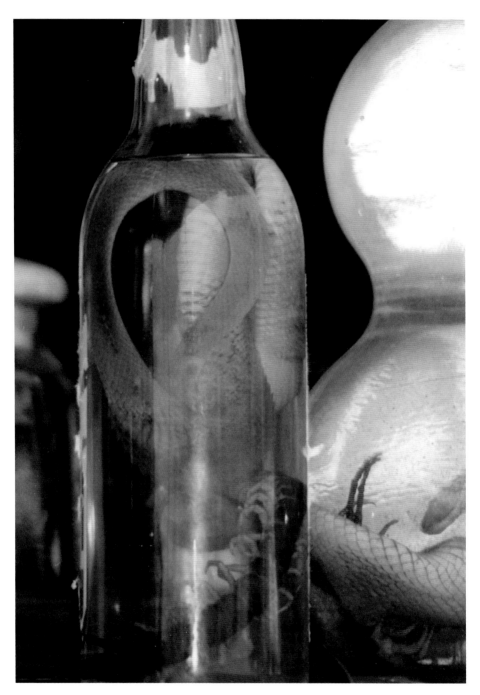

Exotic medicinal drinks are made with poisonous centipedes, snakes, and other insects preserved in alcohol. (Golden Triangle region.)

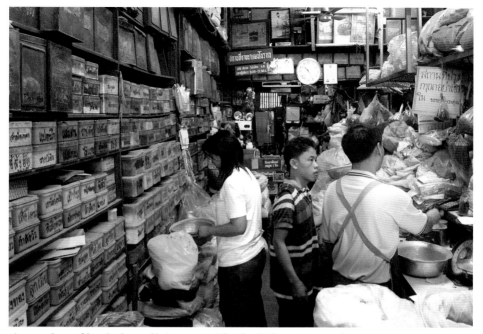

A vendor of herbal medicine outside the Warorot market.

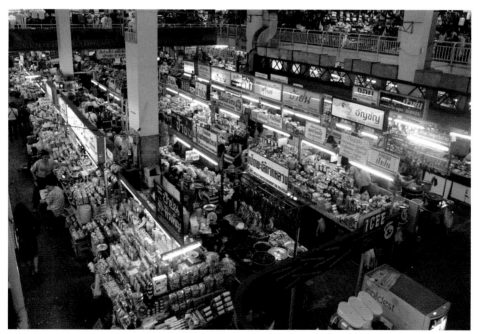

The huge center for herbs and foodstuffs inside Warorot.

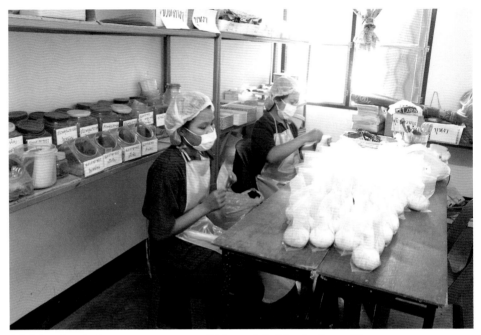

Making herbal compresses at a Chiang Mai herb shop. These women wear masks to avoid inhaling excessive camphor, which is medicinal in small doses but can cause headaches and nausea.

The institution is part of a non-profit charitable endeavor known as the Shivagakomarpaj Foundation, which provides free healthcare to neighboring villages around Chiang Mai on Buddhist holidays. Six times per year, the entire staff—including Western students—piles into vans and heads out into the countryside to treat the villagers with herbs and massage.

Shivagakomarpaj's main focus, however, is as a traditional hospital. Patients are treated with massage, saunas, and traditional herbal remedies by *mo boran* (traditional doctors), and can receive the entire range of traditional Thai therapies under one roof. As mentioned in the introduction, the three branches of Thai medicine are represented in the very architecture of the hospital itself.

The founder of the Old Medicine Hospital was Ajahn Sintorn Chaichakan (Ajahn is an honorific title given to respected teachers, which could be translated as "Master"), who studied traditional Thai medicine at Wat Pho in the late 1950s. Upon completing the degree in 1958, he stayed on as a teacher for four more years. Before that time, Wat Pho did not teach Thai massage, and at the personal request of King Rama IX, Ajahn Sintorn was instrumental in starting the massage program to complement the herbal training Wat Pho had offered for many years.

In 1962, he returned to Chiang Mai and began to practice medicine at small dispensaries on the grounds of several city temples. At this time, the government of Thailand was only interested in supporting Western medicine, and Thai traditions were kept alive by their association with Buddhist institutions. Back in the north of Thailand,

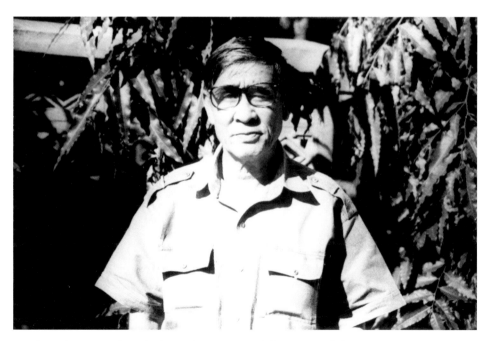

Ajahn Sintorn Chaichakan, director and founder of the Shivagakomarpaj Traditional Medicine Hospital (1962-2005).

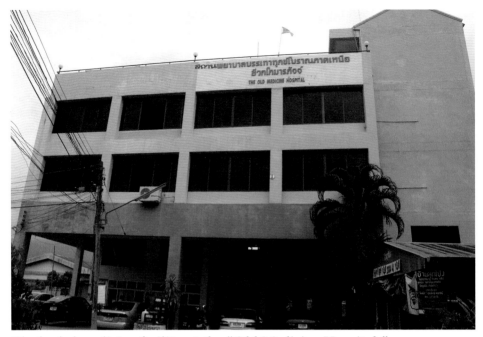

The herbal medicine facility at the "Old Medicine Hospital."

Ajahn Sintorn adapted his practice of massage and herbal medicine to incorporate aspects of northern culture. One important change he made to the Wat Pho massage routine was to slow it down, he says to suit the "laid-back style" of Chiang Mai natives. He also focused on local herbal knowledge, incorporating treatments that were not part of the Wat Pho tradition into his pharmacopoeia.

In 1973, Ajahn Sintorn purchased land just outside of Chiang Mai center and established the current hospital. With only a small grant from the government to start up, the facilities were quite small at that time, with only 10 hospital beds. From these humble beginnings, the hospital grew to the current size. In the 1990s, the program graduated an average of 60-70 Thai students per year in traditional medicine, and the Western students in short courses on Thai massage numbered well into the hundreds.

However, in the last few years, the hospital has lost ground to both Western medical hospitals (several of which have opened up in the city, offering world-class services) and the dozens of less-qualified massage clinics and day spas that have sprung up around Chiang Mai to meet tourist demand. Many of these facilities are unlicensed and staffed by therapists and teachers with little training, and the visitor to Chiang Mai should thus be wary of taking courses or receiving massage outside of the well-known schools. Along with Wat Pho, the Old Medicine Hospital is part of both national and regional efforts to standardize and regulate the massage industry, to improve safety and authenticity of traditional healthcare in the years to come.

Ajahn Sintorn remained the director of the Old Medicine Hospital facility until his passing away on October 19th 2005 and the hospital's affairs are managed today by his sons, Suthat and Wasan. As the next generation assumes control of the hospital's affairs, some changes (such as a new website) have been made to help the hospital compete for students and clients in the modern marketplace. Nonetheless, the Chaichakan family has always prioritized tradition over financial success, and continues to adhere closely to the Thai model of healthcare. Those who are looking for a traditional experience of Thai medicine in a truly authentic environment — whether for study or for a short visit to the sauna — can do no better than the Old Medicine Hospital. Just remember on your way in to stop at the altar and give a wai to Jivaka!

Additional Resources

If you are interested in Chiang Mai, you may want to consult the following materials:

Hargreave, Oliver. Exploring Chiang Mai: City, Valley & Mountains. Chiang Mai: Within Books, 1998. — The most beautiful guidebook I've ever seen for Chiang Mai, as it is full of great photos. It covers the entire region surrounding the city, as well as topics like food and culture.

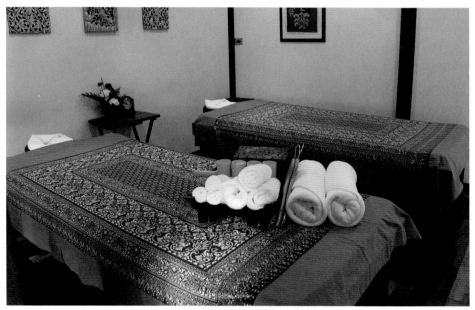

The massage room at a Chiang Mai day spa. These types of facilities appeal to Westerners who are used to luxurious massage clinics back home.

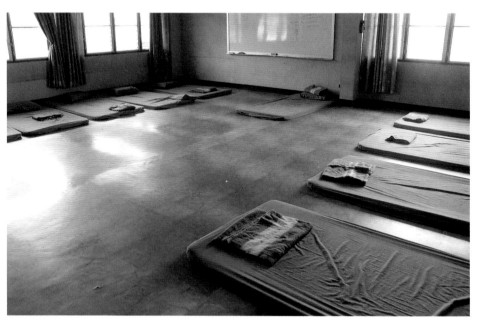

A massage room at Shivagakomarpaj is not as fancy. In traditional Thailand, massage is a part of everyday life, and is usually practiced in a simple communal setting like this.

Lewis, Paul and Elaine. Peoples of the Golden Triangle. Thames and Hudson, Ltd., 1984. - A very informative book on Hill-Tribe customs, with particular focus on material culture. Extensive sections on weaving, silversmithing, and other arts.

www.thaimassageschool.ac.th – The Shivagakomarpaj Traditional Medicine Hospital's website. Check for the English-language link.

www.taomountain.org – Visit my LINKS page to see a continuously-updated list of good massage schools in Chiang Mai, and see the FORUM in the members' area for feedback from students who have recently studied in Thailand.

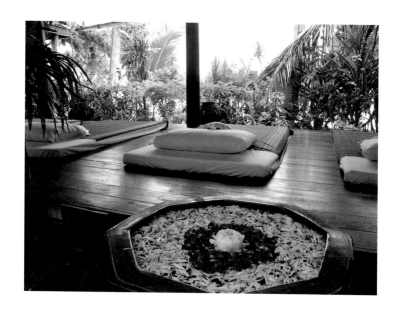

—APPENDIX—

THE TAO MOUNTAIN ASSOCIATION

The Tao Mountain Association is a not-for-profit organization dedicated to the study, preservation, and education of Traditional Thai massage, herbal medicine, healing culture, and Theravada Buddhism. Our organization is focused on supporting teachers and practitioners of Thai healing by providing access to the highest quality of educational materials available in these fields, as well as on charitable activities to give back to the Thai people in gratitude for the wisdom they have shared with us.

Part of the wonderful experience of learning traditional medicine in the country of its origin is the opportunity to participate in a rich blend of ancient culture. One of the most interesting facets of traditional Thai medicine for me is the way in which it has historically intertwined closely with religious and spiritual traditions, and taps into a cultural heritage thousands of years old. When I moved from Thailand back to the U.S. and started teaching Thai massage and herbal medicine, I wanted to provide for my students an experience similar to the one I had during the almost five years I spent living and studying in Southeast Asia.

Westerners obviously have responded enthusiastically to Thai bodywork, but many are unaware of the systematic philosophy of Thai medicine, the uniquely Thai adaptations of Ayurveda, or the practices of Theravada Buddhism and indigenous spiritual traditions—or how these historically and culturally tie into the more familiar Thai healing modalities such as Thai Massage. There is also a tendency to confuse Thai medicine with Chinese medicine or Indian Ayurveda, without taking the tradition on its own terms. The result of this unfortunate situation is that Thai healing traditions are not usually understood as the whole, complete, vibrant indigenous systems that they are. This undermines the existence of Thai medicine as a unique and viable cultural heritage.

I founded Tao Mountain in 2002 as a small school of Thai medicine. One of my primary goals was to share my knowledge of Thai traditions with Western health-care professionals, and to supplement the learning of those who have had the opportunity to live or study abroad with precise and extensive historical, cultural, and theoretical training. Since the beginning, TM's courses, materials, publications, and on-line Resource Center have been geared towards achieving this goal. My goal is to educate and support the best and most authentic teachers of Thai massage and herbal medicine in the industry.

In recent years, the organization has expanded to include a network of teachers who are interested in learning about, preserving, and promoting traditional Thai healing culture. These are Tao Mountain's guiding principles:

- Practitioners and teachers of Thai therapies should be educated in the history, theory, and cultural studies surrounding Thai medicine.
- The traditions of Thai medicine are at the beginning stages of study, and this research into these fields needs to be conducted in an open, collaborative, and mutually non-competitive manner.

- Academic honesty and a spirit of *metta* (or universal kindness), rather than "marketability," should be the driving factors in our research, courses, and personal practices.
- Thai medicine needs to be studied and taught independently of Indian and Chinese traditions, and indigenous Thai traditions need to be emphasized and explored.
- Thai medicine cannot be separated from the spiritual traditions with which it is traditionally bound, and should always be taught with this in mind.
- Thai healing is a medical discipline, and should be studied in this context.

As a not-for-profit organization, Tao Mountain is dedicated to supporting the sharing of knowledge in a fair, equal, non-competitive and intellectually honest manner which will benefit the entire Thai medicine community both in Thailand and abroad. All of our efforts are grounded in an understanding of and respect for authentic Thai tradition. We are also involved in funding charitable projects to give back to the Thai people by promoting traditional healing and healthcare initiatives in rural areas.

Our primary interest is in creating a dialogue between practitioners of Thai healing arts, medical professionals, and academic researchers. We believe that this dialogue is both fruitful and necessary to the continued study of Thai medicine and its many applications in the modern world. Contact us or visit us on-line to see how you can get involved and support this mission as a student, a teacher, or as a general member. Thanks for your help!

— Pierce Salguero

10% of the author's proceeds from sales of this book are given to Tao Mountain's Shivago Fund for use in charitable activities in Thailand, with particular focus on traditional medicine and children's healthcare. A portion of this fund is used to finance the Shivagakomarpaj Traditional Medicine Hospital's village healthcare initiatives described in Chapter 8.

—INDEX—

Other books by C. Pierce Salguero

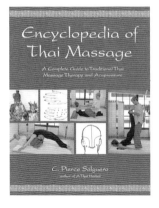
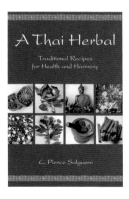

Encyclopedia of Thai Massage:
A Complete Guide to Traditional Thai Massage Therapy and Acupressure

Thai Massage is an increasingly popular healing modality and this book, as its title suggests, is the single most informative and comprehensive book on Thai Massage ever written. With more than 200 full-color photographs and diagrams which beautifully and clearly illustrate the points made in the text, everyone will enjoy and benefit from this unique volume, whatever their level of experience.

250-page paperback, ISBN 1-84409-029-9

A Thai Herbal:
Traditional Recipes for Health and Harmony

Based on the holistic principles of Ayurvedic and traditional Chinese medicine, Thai herbalism is a vibrant ancient tradition, which has been preserved for over a millennium in the monasteries and temples of Bangkok. This book is informative and practical, translating ancient ideas into a modern context and providing helpful tips and recipes for experienced and beginning herbalists.

196-page paperback, ISBN 1-84409-004-3

available from
www.findhornpress.com